GARY W. H. CHANCE

Cancer Highway

A Deadly Journey That Must End

First edition

Contents

Introduction

igarettes represent a public health crisis, with harmful effects extending far beyond those who choose to smoke. Much of the damage inflicted is tolerated by the most vulnerable, those who have never lit a cigarette yet suffer the consequences regardless. *The Cancer Highway* aims to expose smoking for what it is: a killer operating in plain sight, often excused, or overlooked, but leaving a trail of illness, loss, and financial strain in its wake. Cigarettes, far from being harmless personal habits, function as weapons that devastate entire communities. Tolerating their presence should no longer be an option.

The dangers of smoking are well-documented. Despite decades of anti-smoking campaigns, public awareness initiatives, and smoking bans, cigarettes maintain a formidable grip on society. Millions suffer from chronic illnesses like asthma, lung disease, and cancer; all because someone else inconsiderably chose to smoke. So why, in an era of growing health consciousness, does this threat persist? How does the tobacco industry continue to thrive despite widespread knowledge of its dangers?

This book does more than pose questions; it seeks answers through clarity and evidence. It delves into the real-world consequences of smoking, focusing not just on smokers but on innocent bystanders, children, families, co-workers, who are unwilling passengers on this "*Cancer Highway.*" Through vivid examples, staggering statistics, and personal stories, the scope of the damage caused by cigarettes will be explored.

To grasp the magnitude of smoking's impact, it's essential to shift your perspective. Smoking has long been framed as an individual choice, a matter of personal freedom. "It's my body, my choice," some smokers argue. However, this framing ignores a critical fact: cigarettes do not respect boundaries. Their smoke does not remain confined to the person holding the cigarette. Instead, it travels; into the lungs of passers-by, the air around bus stops, the front of shops, schools, offices, restaurants, and homes, you name it. Non-smokers are forced to breathe in harmful chemicals without their consent on a daily basis, there is no escape.

Furthermore, the smoke doesn't simply vanish after a cigarette is extinguished. Toxic particles linger on clothing, furniture, and in the very air that people, particularly children and the elderly, continue to inhale. In workplaces, prior to the implementation of smoking bans, non-smoking employees had no choice but to inhale the same toxic fumes as their smoking colleagues. Although bans have been instituted in many public spaces, anyone can attest to the unpleasantness of working alongside a smoker. When they return from their break, the stench of cigarettes loudly announces the invisible toxins that follow. Everyone in the vicinity have no choice but to breathe in those toxins and live with the consequences.

In outdoor areas where smoking is permitted, bystanders are subjected to second-hand smoke, unable to escape its harmful effects. In *The Cancer Highway*, these uncomfortable truths will be confronted head-on. Smoking is not merely an individual decision; it is a societal issue that harms everyone. Despite overwhelming evidence of the harm caused by cigarettes, they still maintain a stronghold in our culture. Part of this persistence stems from how smoking has been framed and marketed over the years.

This book will outline the physical, emotional, and financial tolls that smoking imposes on non-smokers, emphasizing that no one is truly safe as long as cigarettes exist. It will also navigate the psychological and cultural forces that have kept smoking alive. For decades, the tobacco industry has expertly manipulated public perception, presenting cigarettes as symbols of freedom, rebellion, and sophistication. From James Dean's iconic cigarette-dangling image to today's influencers promoting smoking as a social activity, cigarettes have been glorified and romanticized, obscuring their deadly reality.

Young people are often drawn into smoking not out of a desire for addiction but to fit in, to appear "cool," or to cope with social pressures. This book will dissect these cultural influences, illustrating how they have created fertile ground for nicotine addiction to thrive. By revealing the tricks and tactics employed by the tobacco industry, *The Cancer Highway* will help you see that smoking is not a free choice, but the result of careful manipulation designed to keep people hooked.

As you begin this journey through this book, consider your role in this fight. Whether you are a smoker, a non-smoker, or someone who has lost a loved one to a smoking-related illness, this issue touches all of us. Cigarettes are not just personal vices; they are societal villains. Together, we possess the power to banish them for good. By the end of this book, you will have the tools, knowledge, and motivation to demand change and protect future generations from the dangers of this vile habit.

The road ahead may be difficult, but it is one that we have already been travelling on, whether you stopped to think about it or not. For the sake of health, children, and a smoke-free future, the journey on the *Cancer Highway* must come to an end.

Part 1: Poison in the Air – The Unseen Impact of Second-hand Smoke

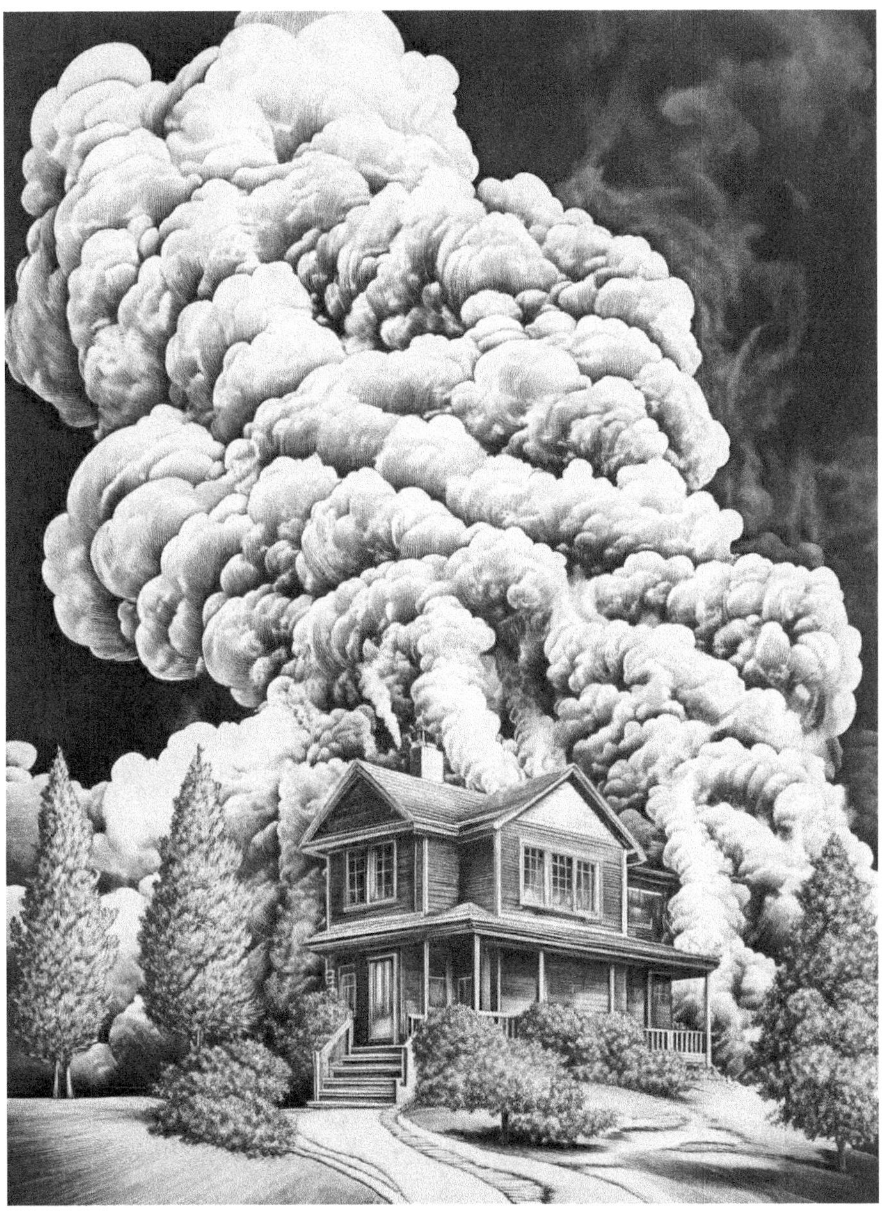

Chapter 1 | Casualties on the Cancer Highway – Diagnosing the Problem

You are driving down a scenic highway on a clear autumn day, with the road stretching smoothly before you and the air crisp and clean. The trees along the roadside are ablaze with vibrant colours, and everything feels open and fresh. But suddenly, the lane ahead becomes clouded with thick, suffocating smoke; dense, acrid, and inescapable. It's as if you've unknowingly driven into a toxic fog, blurring your vision, and clogging your lungs. This sudden change captures the insidious nature of smoking, a destructive force that not only traps the smoker but also veers unsuspecting passers-by into a collision course with its toxic consequences.

In that moment, you realize this isn't just a reckless driver taking a risky detour; it's a highway hazard that threatens everyone on the road. Today, we need to face an uncomfortable truth: cigarette smoke isn't a matter of personal choice; it's a multi-lane pile-up on society's highway, putting innocent lives at risk.

Health Impact on Innocents

Let's dive into a little bit of the science of what a cloud of cigarette smoke is comprised of. A cigarette contains over 7,000 chemicals, of which approximately 250 are harmful and at least 69 are known carcinogens. Just think about that: 7,000 chemicals, burning in a chaotic harmony, caking the insides of your lungs with toxins and polluting the entirety of your system. Among the worst offenders in this hellish concoction of chemicals, there are four specific substances that I think is important to bring more awareness to.

Tar is a sticky substance that builds up in the lungs over time. It is a by-product of burning tobacco and contains numerous toxic chemicals, including those that cause cancer. When a cigarette is smoked, tar collects in the respiratory tract, obstructing air passages and impairing lung function. This accumulation doesn't just sit idly; it gradually transforms the lungs into a breeding ground for chronic respiratory diseases such as chronic obstructive pulmonary disease (COPD) and emphysema.

The long-term effects of tar on the lungs are profoundly damaging and often permanent. When inhaled, the sticky, toxic substance coats the airways and disrupts the function of cilia, the tiny hair-like structures responsible for sweeping away mucus and debris from the respiratory tract. As tar accumulates, the cilia become paralyzed and lose their ability to clear irritants, leading to dangerous stagnation in the lungs. Consequently, chronic coughing, difficulty breathing, and increased susceptibility to infections can follow. Quitting smoking does not end the harm. Tar can persist in the lungs for years, even after the last cigarette is extinguished, leaving behind lasting scars, permanently altering lung tissue, and reducing lung function for the rest of a former smoker's life. This underscores the reality that smoking isn't just a fleeting choice; it's a decision that inflicts long-term damage and increases the risk of debilitating respiratory diseases for the user and those around them.

Next, let's discuss the role formaldehyde plays, a common preservative used in various industrial applications, including the production of building materials and household products, and, as it is mostly well known, for embalming dead bodies. The substance is also present in cigarette smoke as a by-product of combustion. Formaldehyde is classified as a human carcinogen and a potent irritant to the eyes, skin, and respiratory tract.

When inhaled, formaldehyde can cause a range of immediate health issues, including coughing, wheezing, and chest pain. Long-term exposure can lead to more severe respiratory problems, including asthma and chronic bronchitis. Moreover, studies have indicated that formaldehyde exposure can damage lung tissue and affect the immune system's ability to fight infections. This impact on the immune system can leave individuals vulnerable to illnesses that might otherwise be easily manageable.

Benzene is a chemical commonly associated with gasoline fumes and industrial emissions. Benzene is also a notorious component of cigarette smoke and has been linked to various blood cancers, particularly leukaemia.

Benzene disrupts the normal functioning of bone marrow, where blood cells are produced. When benzene enters the bloodstream, it can damage the DNA within these cells, leading to mutations. This genetic alteration increases the risk of cancer, as the body's ability to regulate cell growth is compromised. The effects of benzene exposure are not immediate; they may take years to manifest, which is why its presence in cigarette smoke is so insidious. Chronic exposure can also lead to a condition known as aplastic anaemia, where the bone marrow fails to produce enough blood cells, resulting in fatigue, increased susceptibility to infections, and excessive bleeding.

To recover from aplastic anaemia, treatment options vary based on the patient's health and circumstances. A bone marrow transplant (BMT) is the most definitive curative treatment but requires a matched donor and may not be suitable for everyone. For patients who cannot undergo a transplant, immunosuppressive therapy using drugs like antithymocyte globulin (ATG), and cyclosporine can help restore bone marrow function and achieve long-term remission in many cases. Additionally, blood transfusions may be necessary to manage low blood counts, and medications that stimulate blood cell production can further support recovery.

Lastly, I want to discuss carbon monoxide (CO), a colourless, odourless gas that is a by-product of burning tobacco. Carbon monoxide is particularly dangerous because it binds to haemoglobin in the blood, this is the molecule responsible for transporting oxygen throughout the body. In fact, carbon monoxide binds to haemoglobin with an affinity 200 times greater than oxygen, in simpler words, your blood cells, when they have to choose between oxygen and carbon monoxide, they will choose the latter 200 times over before they even consider the oxygen, put that in perspective. When carbon monoxide is present, it effectively hijacks the oxygen-carrying capacity of the blood. As a result, less oxygen is available to vital organs and tissues, leading to a condition known as hypoxia. Hypoxia can cause symptoms such as shortness of breath, dizziness, and confusion. Over time, inadequate oxygen supply can lead to severe cardiovascular issues, including heart disease and stroke.

For individuals with pre-existing health conditions, the effects can be even more pronounced. Those with heart disease, for instance, may experience angina (chest pain) or heart attacks as their hearts struggle to pump enough oxygen-rich blood to meet the body's demands. The cumulative effects of carbon monoxide can thus lead to a gradual decline in overall health and a significantly reduced quality of life.

The Gravity of Cigarette Smoke

Each of these chemicals; tar, formaldehyde, benzene, and carbon monoxide; paints a picture of the toxic landscape created by smoking. It is not just a habit; it is an act that endangers both the smoker and those around them. The scientific reality is clear: smoking is not an isolated personal choice; it has far-reaching consequences that ripple through individuals and communities.

As we learn more about these chemicals, their interactions, and their devastating effects, we must confront the uncomfortable truth: tolerating this habit is to put ourselves in danger of inhaling these chemicals with far more frequency than it should ever be acceptable. It is a call to action, an imperative to protect ourselves and our loved ones from the dangers of smoking and second-hand smoke.

Some people might say these extreme health issues are just "worst case" scenarios and that they've never met anyone who's faced such serious conditions. While that's true, it doesn't change the fact that the effects of smoking are progressive. There's a spectrum of harm that goes from bad to worse, with no safe spot in between. From the first moment you inhale cigarette smoke, whether you're the one smoking or just caught in the cloud, you're stepping back toward a negative outcome. Each puff causes damage that most likely will never be reversible.

It's tough to navigate life without inhaling toxic fumes in our modern world. The conveniences we enjoy come with real downsides, many of which are hard to escape. Still, there's no need to hold onto a habit that only brings harm. Smoking is entirely unnecessary today, especially when information about its dangers is so widely available. You don't have to smoke, and you definitely shouldn't have to deal with the consequences of someone else's choices as a passive smoker.

But let's talk a little bit more about the collateral damage for the victims that everyone seems to be willingly ignoring, the children, the non-smokers bystanders who never consented to this risk and are largely incapable to understand or avoid the risks they are put on. As someone who grew up in a household enveloped in smoke, I witnessed the long-lasting effects first-hand. My brother was born "blue," struggling for breath, a direct consequence of my parents' smoking.

Cyanosis is what you call it when a new-born has a bluish tint to their skin, especially around the lips and fingertips. This condition usually indicates that the baby might not be getting enough oxygen, and it can happen for a few reasons, especially if the mother smoked during pregnancy. When a mother smokes, carbon monoxide levels in her blood go up, making it harder for oxygen to reach the foetus, which can lead to hypoxia, or low oxygen levels in the tissues. Nicotine doesn't help either; it tightens blood vessels, cutting down on blood flow and oxygen delivery.

On top of that, congenital heart defects are more common in babies born to moms who smoke, which can mess with the heart's ability to pump oxygenated blood. New-borns can also experience respiratory issues, like meconium aspiration syndrome, which can lead to cyanosis. Prematurity and low birth weight, both often tied to maternal smoking, can increase the chances of these complications.

Many children like my brother are lucky to survive, but countless others are not so fortunate. Children exposed to second-hand smoke are two to three times more likely to develop respiratory infections and asthma. They are set up for a lifetime of struggles, cognitive delays, learning disabilities, and a reduced quality of life.

Imagine the contrasting paths of a child raised in a smoke-filled environment versus one who grows up in a smoke-free home. The former is often more susceptible to sickness, underperforming at school, likely to even develop chronic conditions related to being a passive smoker. They battle not only physical health issues but also emotional scars, watching their peers outperform them. In contrast, the latter thrives, experiencing life without the weight of debilitating respiratory problems. This is not just anecdotal; research shows that children raised in smoke-free homes perform better academically and socially, illustrating the profound impact of environment on childhood development.

When it comes to pregnant women living with smokers, the statistics are sobering. Pregnant women exposed to second-hand smoke are at a higher risk of miscarriage, up to 23% higher, complications during pregnancy, and stillbirth. The emotional toll of miscarriage is indescribable. It's a heart-wrenching experience that leaves a scar far deeper than the physical loss to the mother and to those close to them. Miscarriages related to smoking often feel like a betrayal of the body, a crushing blow that erases hope in an instant. For every woman, the loss of a child, even before birth, is a devastating experience, often accompanied by feelings of guilt and grief that linger long after, if not forever.

Consider the implications for both mother and baby. Babies born to mothers who smoke during pregnancy are more likely to have low birth weights, which can lead to a myriad of health problems. Moreover, exposure to second-hand smoke during pregnancy can result in lifelong consequences for the child, like developmental issues, increased risk of sudden infant death syndrome (SIDS), and a higher likelihood of becoming smokers themselves later in life.

Globally, over 1 million babies die each year as a result of maternal smoking, with a significant portion of these deaths attributable to second-hand smoke exposure during pregnancy. It's a harsh reality: those who are meant to protect the most vulnerable are sometimes the very source of their harm.

Let's look at the bigger picture through the lens of staggering statistics for passive smokers. At the time of writing this book, In the United States, the Centers for Disease Control and Prevention (CDC) reports that approximately 41,000 non-smokers die each year from second-hand smoke exposure. In the UK, the figure is around 12,000 deaths annually. Globally, the World Health Organization (WHO) estimates that second-hand smoke contributes to the deaths of more than 890,000 people each year. These figures aren't just numbers; they represent lives cut short, families torn apart, and communities forever changed.

Just so you are also aware, these statistics when related to the smoker themselves are, in the United States, approximately 480,000 deaths, with 16 million Americans living disease caused by smoking. Across the pond, in the UK, smoking accounts for 74,600 annual deaths and globally, that number skyrockets to 8 million people. These deaths are slow, painful, frustrating and utterly avoidable.

Mental Health: A Silent Suffering

The impact on mental health is an often-overlooked aspect of second-hand smoke. Breathing in cigarette smoke, especially in shared spaces; homes, workplaces, or public areas, can create an atmosphere of anxiety and powerlessness among non-smokers. Imagine you're sitting at the park, just having your lunch break, when someone next to you lights a cigarette. The air that was fresh a moment ago now feels heavy and sharp, and you can't help but breathe in the acrid smoke. Your throat gets scratchy, your eyes sting, and it's not just uncomfortable; it's irritating. You didn't choose this, but now you're stuck inhaling someone else's habit, wishing you could escape that lingering cloud.

This discomfort can lead to increased stress and anxiety levels. The American Psychological Association highlights that environments filled with second-hand smoke can contribute to a decline in overall mental well-being. The psychological toll is exacerbated when individuals find themselves in social situations, feeling obligated to tolerate the smell and the discomfort rather than risking social faux pas. It becomes a daily struggle, balancing the desire for social interaction with the need for personal well-being.

But the issue isn't just limited to standing in a smoke-filled area. Many smokers don't realize that the lingering smell on their clothes, hair, skin and breath isn't just unpleasant; it's toxic. Breathing in those stale fumes can be just as harmful as direct smoke exposure. Non-smokers in these situations experience the same discomfort, stress, and anxiety, feeling trapped in that invisible cloud of toxins.

Living in a smoke-filled environment is a constant inconvenience. The smell doesn't just stick to the smoker; it clings to everything around them, from other people's clothes to shared spaces and even the furniture. The worst part is that the lingering odour becomes part of you, an unwanted layer that turns even the simplest social interactions into uncomfortable experiences. It creates a kind of social exclusion. How often have you walked into a room and sensed the silent discomfort of non-smokers, forced to breathe in toxins while trying to stay polite?

Chapter 2 | Nowhere to Hide – The Spaces Where Non-Smokers Suffer

Imagine trying to avoid breathing in polluted air while standing on the edge of a freeway. That's how it feels for millions of non-smokers who, despite their best efforts, are forced to inhale toxic smoke in places where they should feel safe, at home, at work, or in public spaces. For these unwilling passengers, there is often no escape from the dangers of smoking. And the worst part? They never volunteered for this ride.

In the previous chapter, we touched on the harsh reality of being an unwilling passenger on the *Cancer Highway*, a journey that non-smokers are forced to take without their consent. We discussed some of the negative effects faced by those who have no choice but to inhale second-hand smoke. And really, "negative effects" being a tautology, because when it comes to second-hand smoke, there's nothing positive in sight. But there's more to uncover here, especially when it comes to how passive smokers are often ignored in this conversation. I want to expand the discussion on this side of the topic. Society has plenty of campaigns, warnings, and labels aimed at smokers, but where's the focus on the people who suffer alongside them? The reality is, non-smokers are often left out of the narrative, despite bearing the brunt of the impact, and it's time to change that.

When people think about the risks of smoking, the focus is often on the smoker alone. But the reality is that the harm radiates far beyond the cigarette's glowing tip. Toxic particles linger in the air, seep through walls, stick to clothes, and settle on surfaces, exposing non-smokers to dangerous chemicals they never consented to breathe. And whether it's your house mate's cigarette smoke drifting through the walls of your apartment, a co-worker taking yet another break to light up, or even just sitting at a park bench while someone smokes nearby, there's an overwhelming sense that there's nowhere to hide.

At Home - A Breathing Battle

For non-smokers, the home is supposed to be a refuge, a place where you can let your guard down, relax, and simply breathe easy. But for many, especially those living with smokers or surrounded by them, that idea is a fantasy. You see, even when smokers think they're being considerate by stepping outside to light up, the poison doesn't just vanish into thin air. The truth is, the toxins cling to clothing, hair, furniture, and walls, creating an invisible threat right in your living room and throughout the house. It's called *third-hand smoke,* and it lingers long after the cigarette is put out.

Most people think of smoking risks as a choice, and sure, for those who choose to smoke, that's true to a point. But let's go into the uncomfortable zone: smoking harms everyone in the smoker's orbit, and despite any smoker's best intentions, the smoke can be undeniably sneaky and insidious. Third-hand smoke is like a toxic ghost, it remains in the air, on surfaces, and in fabrics, even when no one's actively smoking. Imagine it as invisible residue that settles over everything, slowly contaminating your home with harmful chemicals like the substances I expanded on chapter 1 plus others like nicotine, and even lead.

Let me paint a picture for you. A smoker steps outside to take a few puffs. The cigarette burns, releasing thousands of chemicals into the air. They finish up, put out the cigarette, and walk back inside, attached to them, the *third-hand smoke* ghost. When they walk through the front door, so do the toxins.

It sounds dramatic, but it's true. Studies have shown that third-hand smoke can remain detectable in homes for up to six months after a smoker quits. Anyone, more specifically, any non-smoker who visits the house of a smoker can tell of this presence that the smoker and those living in that environment are likely to dismiss. If you've ever visited a smoker's house as a non-smoker, you've likely felt that invisible presence. I've experienced it first-hand with a family member who smokes. She insists she never smokes inside, and maybe that's true, but the unmistakable scent of third-hand smoke clings to the air, furniture, and everything else. Every time we leave, our clothes carry it with us, even into our car. She doesn't seem to notice, but we do the moment we step inside her house.

It's easy to dismiss the effects of third-hand smoke as minor, but here's where it gets real. For kids, it's especially dangerous. Think about how children interact with their environment. They're touching everything, putting their hands in their mouths, playing on the floor, and breathing in more air per pound of body weight than adults. That means every bit of that toxic residue becomes a potential threat to their developing lungs and immune systems.

Now, if you're a non-smoker living with someone who smokes, this might all sound terrifying, especially because you are experiencing that effect over and over again every day you spend living in that environment. And you're right to be concerned. But you're not alone. I've heard countless stories from non-smokers who are forced to pay the price for someone else's habit.

Consider a couple of scenarios. Lisa, a university student sharing a house with three other roommates. One of them, Ben, is a heavy smoker. Although he promises to only smoke outside, every time he comes back in, the smell of smoke lingers on his clothes and hair, trailing into the shared living spaces. The situation is even worse when friends visit and light up on the back patio, thinking that it's far enough away. The house's poor ventilation lets the smoke creep into Lisa's room and the common areas. Over time, Lisa began to suffer from chronic bronchitis, persistent coughing, and a wheeze that wouldn't go away. The sad part? She never once chose to smoke, but her health has paid the price for someone else's choice.

Or John, a father raising two young children. His neighbour frequently smoked at the back of his house, just a few feet away from the children's bedroom window. John kept the windows closed when possible, thinking it would keep the smoke out. But even with the windows shut tight, the toxic particles still managed to find their way inside. His children, both under five, began waking up with scratchy throats and stuffy noses. They hadn't signed up for this; John hadn't signed up for this either. And yet, there they were, breathing in someone else's poison.

And that's just the human side of the story. The numbers back it up too. In the USA, the CDC has reported that even brief exposure to second-hand smoke can damage the lining of blood vessels and increase the risk of heart disease. It's not just a casual whiff here or there, it's about long-term consequences. When the toxins are settling in your home, you're facing a constant low-level exposure that chips away at your health over time.

You wouldn't be casually walking down the corridors of the Chernobyl power plant, would you? Even though a large area around the plant has been deemed "safe", there is still a very low exposure that if experienced constantly, will cause harm. The same is happening with low-level exposures to cigarette smoke.

Now, let's zoom out for a moment and think about the bigger picture. For our American readers for example, if you live in an apartment or multi-unit building, your exposure risk goes up. The ventilation systems in these buildings aren't airtight; they're designed to circulate air, which means that toxic particles can easily travel between units. You could be living next door to a heavy smoker and not even know it, yet you're still breathing in the residue of their habit every single day. It's a sobering thought, and it's not just paranoia, it's a fact supported by research.

But it's not just about shared spaces. It's about shared air. Even in single-family homes, the toxins don't stay confined to one room. Studies have shown that third-hand smoke particles can move through the air and attach to surfaces throughout an entire house, including areas where no one has smoked. This is particularly concerning if you have children, elderly family members, or anyone with respiratory issues living with you. And here's the kicker, it doesn't matter if the smoker thinks they're being careful. It doesn't matter if they always go outside or crack a window. Those toxins are persistent, and they don't need an invitation to spread.

It's frustrating because, for non-smokers, there's no real choice in the matter. You don't get to choose the air you breathe when you live with a smoker or next door to one. The consequences are imposed on you, and often, it feels like there's nowhere to hide. Your home, your sanctuary, becomes a toxic battleground, and you didn't even sign up for the fight.

So, what can you do? First, if you live with a smoker, start by having an honest conversation. Insist on a strict, genuine no-smoking policy, both inside and outside the house. It might feel like a tough demand, but it's not unreasonable to ask for clean air in your own home. Advocate for stronger regulations in multi-unit housing. Push for smoke-free policies that protect not just the residents who choose to smoke but also those who don't have that choice. The laws are moving in this direction, but until they catch up, it's on you to protect your space. If we must consider the worst-case scenario, simply move away if you can, your health should be one of your top priorities, because it dictates how long and the quality of life you live.

If you're the smoker, I'm not here to demonize you. Quitting is hard, I get that. But know this: your choices don't just affect you. They ripple out and impact the people you love, even if they never pick up a cigarette themselves. It's not about judgment; it's about responsibility. We all share the air we breathe, and we have a duty to protect each other from harm. By cultivating such habits, you are personally imposing a negative effect on the health of those around you, even if you are trying to do your best to prevent that. This is hard to hear, but there is no other way to put it bluntly.

So, here's the bottom line: your home should be a place of safety and health, not a battlefield against invisible toxins. If you're a non-smoker dealing with this, take action. Speak up, set boundaries, and demand the clean air you deserve. If you're a smoker, consider the impact of your choices on those around you. Think about the silent harm you might be causing, even if you can't see it. At the end of the day, everyone has the right to breathe easy in their own home. No one should be forced to inhale cancer-causing toxins or deal with the myriad of health issues that come with second-hand or third-hand smoke.

When it comes to smoking in our homes, there really is nowhere to hide from the damage. The impact is real, and the consequences are lasting. And that's not just my opinion, it's the truth backed by science and the stories of countless people who never chose this fight.

In the Workplace - Trapped in Toxicity

Workplaces are supposed to be environments of productivity, collaboration, and personal growth. Yet for years, many became silent battlegrounds in an ongoing fight against smoking habits. Millions of workers unknowingly inhale harmful toxins every day, simply trying to earn a living.

In the past, employees in bars, restaurants, and other public spaces faced the highest levels of second-hand smoke exposure, because if you don't know or don't remember, it was legal to smoke at work or indoors. Think about that: serving drinks, cleaning tables, cooking meals, or managing customers while clouds of smoke lingered in the air. People spent hours inside environments like that, breathing it in, they went home each day with a stench so heavy in their clothes and hair that it became part of their identity, whether they wanted it or not. Thirty or Forty years ago, this was so common that people were used to the smell of it, most would hardly notice it. Their workplaces were basically filled with invisible smoke-filled walls, and the reality was, many had no choice but to endure it to keep their jobs. It's not a matter of the past, either. Even today, where smoking bans have significantly reduced exposure in many countries, the risk remains in less regulated areas or places where bans are not enforced strictly.

Take a moment to imagine it, working alongside someone who repeatedly takes smoke breaks, returning to the office reeking of toxins. It's not just the smell; like we discussed previously, it's the lingering chemicals that follow them back in. There's something particularly frustrating about being at your desk, focused on your tasks, only to be interrupted by someone's smoke residue infiltrating your space. Each break might take just a few minutes, but that is enough to cause prolonged discomfort and negative effects to the health of those around smokers. These non-smokers are still involuntarily exposed to second-hand and third-hand smoke, and no amount of air fresheners or open windows can truly shield them from that. Today, it is not legal to smoke indoors, and the majority of places enforce that, at least most places and countries I have been myself, but that didn't solve the problem exactly when someone go away to smoke to immediately come back to impose the effects of it on those who don't smoke.

I'm not only against that habit, I'm actually allergic to the habit. I can detect smokers a mile away, I can tell the smallest traces of it in an environment because it triggers an allergic reaction in me. I have worked in places where colleagues had a habit of going out for multiple breaks throughout their shifts for a "fag" as we call in the UK. They would come back in and immediately trigger a reaction in me, it was very frustrating and I have always been vocal about it, to my own detriment. Smokers will firmly defend their habit, "I went outside to smoke", it doesn't matter if I'm allergic or inconvenienced by it, the law is on their side and it doesn't batter an eye lid towards people like me, because for the lawmakers, the harm magically ends with the last puff.

To make matters worse, consider the disparity in treatment between smokers and non-smokers in workplaces. Think about it. Smokers often get frequent breaks, sometimes even as a group or in pairs, stepping outside to indulge their habit, while non-smokers are expected to remain at their desks, productive and efficient, without similar allowances. How many times have non-smokers watched a colleague stroll out for a smoke break, returning after 10 minutes while they continued working without pause? Not only is this a health issue, but it's a workplace fairness issue as well. Non-smokers does not only have to tolerate it, but also have to endure the toxic slap-on-the-face every time it happens.

For those in customer-facing roles like waiters and bartenders, the impact has been even more severe. Before smoking bans became widespread, these workers faced hours of direct exposure each day. In fact, studies from that period showed that workers in smoke-filled environments had a significantly higher risk of lung cancer and heart disease compared to other professions.

And even now, in some countries where regulations are still weak or not well enforced, the situation hasn't changed much.

Think of Tom, a bartender in a busy pub back in the early 1990's. Every shift meant eight hours or more of standing amidst clouds of cigarette smoke. He never smoked a single cigarette in his life, but by the time he was in his thirties, Tom's doctor diagnosed him with chronic bronchitis and early signs of emphysema. Years of inhaling second-hand smoke behind the bar had taken a toll on his lungs. Tom's story isn't unique. Thousands of hospitality workers suffered similar fates, forced to choose between their income and their health.

Although the scenario above is much rarer today, in countries that enforces strong regulations, we still deal with a level of the same perils through second and third-hand smoke. I am always upset to see chefs and kitchen staff taking smoking breaks, sometime mere steps from their workstation. People who are cooking the food that we eat. Such workplace must follow strict health and safety regulations that can cost them their license or a hefty fine when broken, yet everyone seems to be blind that the staff is handling other people's food inside a 700 plus chemicals toxic cloud that emanate from their bodies after every smoke break.

The effects of second-hand and third-hand smoke don't vanish with the implementation of smoking bans or any of the smoke regulations we have in place today. For those who work outdoors or in shared public spaces, the risk continues. Think of the delivery driver constantly driving and walking by smokers on the street. Or the janitor cleaning an outdoor event space after hours of attendees smoking at tables. Even in "regulated" environments, enforcement of smoke-free laws often fails to protect the most vulnerable.

And beyond just the physical toll, there's an emotional and mental burden to bear. Working alongside someone who brings the stench of smoke back from breaks can create a tense atmosphere. You're not just forced to endure the toxins; you're also placed in an uncomfortable social situation. Do you speak up and risk being seen as difficult? Or do you stay silent and deal with the daily impact on your health?

For those who have asthma, allergies, or respiratory issues, the situation is even worse. The irritation caused by third-hand smoke can trigger symptoms and lead to frequent health issues, turning a regular workday into a struggle just to breathe.

Despite all of this, it's still easy for people to brush off these concerns. "It's not like anyone's smoking inside," some might say. But we already know that smoke doesn't respect boundaries. A smoke break outside doesn't mean the toxins stay outside. And just because there's a sign banning smoking indoors doesn't mean the effects disappear once the cigarette is out.

If you're in a position of authority at work, it's your responsibility to set the tone. Make your workplace genuinely smoke-free, inside and out. Protect not just the smokers trying to quit but the non-smokers who have no choice but to breathe in the lingering consequences of other people's habits. And for the smokers reading this, remember that quitting isn't just about your health. It's about the well-being of your co-workers, the people you share your space with every single day. Your choices impact more than just you.

At the end of the day, no one should have to put their health on the line just to earn a living. Everyone deserves a workplace where they can breathe easily, without the threat of second-hand or third-hand smoke. We've made strides in creating healthier work environments, but there's still a long road ahead. It's not just about laws and regulations; it's about fostering a culture where people's well-being takes priority over outdated habits. Because at work, just like anywhere else, there should be no room for cancer-causing toxins. Work shouldn't be a place where you have to choose between your health and your pay check. It should be a place where you can thrive, not suffocate. And that's the bottom line.

In Public Spaces - The Relentless Reach of Smoke

Imagine standing at a bus stop, waiting for your ride to arrive. You're minding your business, maybe scrolling through your phone or enjoying the fresh air. Suddenly, someone nearby lights up a cigarette. Instantly, the air around you changes; heavy, sharp, and inescapable. You're now stuck between staying in this toxic cloud or moving farther down the street, risking missing your bus altogether. And here's the thing: this isn't a rare occurrence. This is everyday life for millions of non-smokers who find themselves in public spaces, just trying to get through their day.

Parks, sidewalks, beaches, bus stops, these are places where you should be able to relax or pass through without a second thought. But for non-smokers, especially those with respiratory issues, these public spaces are often filled with unexpected threats. It's a frustrating situation. You want to enjoy a day out with your kids, but you find yourself surrounded by people puffing away at park benches or near playgrounds. You're trying to take a jog, breathe deeply, and clear your mind, only to hit a pocket of lingering smoke that burns your throat and stings your eyes. This is not just an inconvenience. It's a health hazard that many have no choice but to endure. It's as if no matter where you go, you're always trying to escape someone else's smoke.

When people hear the term "second-hand smoke," they often think of indoor spaces; homes, offices, bars. But outdoor spaces can be just as dangerous. Smoke doesn't simply vanish into thin air. It lingers, drifts, and clings to people. A 2016 study by Stanford University found that even in open-air environments, a person standing within a few feet of a smoker can inhale significant amounts of harmful toxins. Think about that. Even outdoors, you're still at risk.

It's not just about an unpleasant smell or temporary irritation. For those with asthma, allergies, or other respiratory issues, even brief exposure to cigarette smoke, yes, even outdoors, can trigger symptoms like shortness of breath, coughing, sneezing, and wheezing. And this isn't just discomfort; it's a real health threat. Imagine a parent taking their children to the local playground for a fun afternoon. Other parents are there too, and one of them decides to light a cigarette nearby. The smoke drifts over, and suddenly, what was supposed to be a carefree day turns into a struggle to breathe. Children and parents are left suffering because of a decision they didn't make. Non-smokers pay the price, and an innocent outing is ruined by someone else's choice.

This brings up an uncomfortable question: Why should non-smokers be the ones forced to adjust? Why should the burden of finding clean air fall on them? There's a misconception that smoking is a personal habit, but when that habit starts to infringe on the health of others, it becomes a public issue. Public spaces should be safe for everyone, not just the people who choose to light up.

Some people argue that public smoking bans infringe on personal freedom. But here's the thing: freedom shouldn't come at the cost of someone else's well-being. Everyone has the right to access public spaces without being exposed to toxins. When your personal habit starts to harm others, it's no longer just about you. It's about the collective right to breathe clean air.

And let's talk about children for a moment. Kids don't get a say in where they're exposed to smoke. When parents or other adults smoke around them, children are forced to inhale toxic fumes, their developing lungs paying the price. According to the CDC, children exposed to second-hand smoke have increased risks of ear infections, severe asthma attacks, and respiratory infections. The worst offenders are the parents who will smoke around their children, at home, inside their cars or even outdoors, exposing that child to severe second and third-hand smoke.

What's even more troubling is that children who grow up around smokers are more likely to become smokers themselves. They see smoking as normal, something adults do in parks, at beaches, or while waiting for buses. It's a learned behaviour, one that perpetuates the cycle of addiction and harm. So, when we allow smoking in public spaces, we're not just affecting people's immediate health; we're also setting up future generations to suffer the same fate. I myself have experienced that desire when I was a child, my parents were smokers, I always imagined myself growing up and smoking like them. I remember asking my parents if I could even try it every now and then (to which they always said no). Unknowingly to everyone, just living in that environment, I was already cultivating a habit of smoking by association. Luckily, I grew up to despise the habit as my brother didn't.

Some cities have started to catch on. San Francisco, for example, banned smoking at all bus stops and in public parks back in 2010, setting a precedent for others to follow. But even with these strides, enforcement is often weak, and the rules aren't consistent across different regions. In some places, it feels like public smoking bans are just suggestions, with little to no consequences for those who ignore them.

There's also the issue of what happens to the places that are supposed to be safe. Beaches and parks often have designated smoking areas, but these zones aren't contained. The smoke drifts, carried by the breeze, affecting everyone nearby. You might think you're far enough away from the designated smoking area, but I don't have to remind you, smoke knows no boundaries. It travels, sometimes farther than you might think.

If you've ever tried to relax on a beach towel, only to have a cloud of smoke blow over from a nearby group, you know the frustration. Beaches, which should be havens of fresh air and open spaces, can easily turn into smoky battlegrounds where you're constantly trying to escape an invisible threat. And it's not just a nuisance; it's a risk to your health.

And then there are places like the bus stop example we gave earlier. A place where, let's be honest, you're kind of trapped. You can't exactly walk away without risking missing your bus or train. It's a captive audience situation, and smokers don't care. You've probably seen it before: someone lights up, and now everyone else is stuck breathing in their smoke. This creates a dynamic where non-smokers are left holding their breath, trying to edge away while feeling frustrated and helpless.

Ultimately, this isn't just about inconvenience or irritation. It's about health, fairness, and the right to clean air. Public spaces should belong to everyone, and no one should have to sacrifice their well-being just to go about their day. We've made progress in addressing smoking in indoor spaces, but we're still falling short when it comes to protecting non-smokers in public areas. The solutions are there: stronger enforcement, clearer regulations, and a shift in public attitudes.

If you're reading this as a smoker, you might feel defensive or even attacked, but consider this: the choice to smoke is impacting others in ways you might not have realized. It's not just a personal decision when it infringes on someone else's health, it becomes my problem when I have to breathe-in your bad habit. And if you're a non-smoker, it's time to stop accepting this as the status quo. Speak up, advocate for smoke-free spaces, and demand the right to breathe clean air.

Public spaces should be safe for everyone. That means not having to dodge clouds of smoke just to walk your dog, enjoy a picnic, or wait for the bus. It means recognizing that smoking isn't just a habit, it's a public health issue with far-reaching consequences. And it means standing up for your right to breathe easy, no matter where you are.

Chapter 3 | The Financial Fallout – How Smoking Hurts Everyone

When you think of the negative points of smoking, what comes to mind? Maybe the classic warnings about lung cancer or the lingering stench of the habit. Most people understand that smoking is harmful to the individual smoker. Most people also understand about just how deeply it hurts everyone else around too, even though it is wildly ignored. But I want to highlight another side of it too, I'm talking about the hidden financial costs and the emotional toll that stretch far beyond those who light up. The truth is, smoking is an expensive habit, not just for those buying the cigarettes, but for entire societies that pay the price in more ways than you might think.

Every time someone smokes, there's a cost that echoes throughout the entire community. It's not just the price of a pack of cigarettes, but the burden on healthcare systems, the losses faced by businesses, and the emotional weight carried by families. If you think about it, smoking is a drain on resources in ways that are often subtle and unspoken.

This chapter isn't just about numbers and statistics, though those are essential to understanding the scope of the problem. It's about shedding light on a reality that many of us don't see or don't want to acknowledge.

Because when we focus solely on the health impacts of smoking, we miss the bigger picture: the systemic ways in which smoking costs everyone; smokers, non-smokers, employers, families, and entire nations. Let's dive into that idea a bit further.

Healthcare Burden

Let's talk about a different cost of the smoking habit, a cost that goes far beyond the price of a pack of cigarettes or the health of the individual smoker. The financial burden that smoking places on healthcare systems isn't just a line item on a budget report; it's a reflection of lives lost, resources drained, and priorities skewed in the face of preventable harm. When we think about the impact of smoking, we have to start looking at it through a wider lens. Because smoking isn't just a personal vice, it's a public crisis that burdens entire healthcare systems and siphons away billions of dollars each year.

In the United States alone, smoking-related diseases cost the healthcare system around $225 billion annually. Think about that figure for a second. That's a massive weight on an already-strained system, pulling resources away from other critical needs and overburdening hospitals, clinics, and the medical professionals who work there. We're talking about funds that could be spent on preventative care, better equipment, or even life-saving research. Instead, those dollars are diverted to treat conditions that, in many cases, never needed to exist in the first place.

The numbers in the UK, while scaled to a smaller population, paint an equally troubling picture. The National Health Service (NHS) spends billions every year dealing with the fallout from smoking. This strain isn't just felt financially, it impacts the quality of care that patients receive, the allocation of resources, and the availability of essential services. The ripple effects extend far beyond the smoker in the hospital bed; they reach into the lives of every citizen who relies on that system.

Likely the USA and the UK, your country also spends a huge amount of its annual budget just dealing with the devastating damages caused by smoke, money that could be better invested in education, health improvements and infrastructure. What other industry out there that you know is solely responsible for only causing harm with absolutely no benefit to the individual and the population and at the same time, solely responsible for draining so much money from the public funds?

You see, when we think about the healthcare costs of smoking, we often picture direct expenses, treating lung cancer, heart disease, and chronic obstructive pulmonary disease (COPD). And yes, these are major financial drains. But smoking doesn't just impact the lungs or the heart. It's a major contributor to conditions like diabetes, rheumatoid arthritis, and even certain types of blindness. Each of these illnesses requires ongoing care, hospital stays, and medications, all adding to the growing financial burden.

But it's not just about hospital bills and medication costs. The strain extends to insurance premiums and the overall economics of healthcare. Here's a harsh reality: everyone, not just smokers, ends up paying more. Insurance companies aren't absorbing those healthcare costs, they're passing them on to policyholders. So, even if you've never touched a cigarette in your life, you're still footing the bill for a crisis created by the tobacco industry. In fact, increased healthcare premiums are a hidden tax on all of us, indirectly subsidizing a deadly habit that we didn't choose to be part of.

Employers feel the sting too. Studies have shown that smokers take more sick days than non-smokers, costing businesses billions annually in lost productivity. It's not just about the occasional smoke break; it's the cumulative impact of increased absences, reduced performance, and the healthcare costs associated with treating smoking-related illnesses. When businesses lose money, they have to make up for it somewhere, which often means higher prices for goods and services or cuts in other areas. And once again, we all end up paying the price.

Now, you might be wondering: Why should I care? Why does it matter if healthcare systems are strained or businesses are losing money? The answer is simple, because these systems are interconnected. When healthcare resources are diverted to treat preventable illnesses, everyone feels the impact. Think of it like a domino effect. A smoker gets hospitalized for a heart attack or emphysema. The hospital devotes time, beds, and staff to treating that patient.

Those resources aren't infinite. They're being taken away from other patients who also need care. The financial burden doesn't just fall on governments or insurance companies, it falls on the public.

Here's where it gets even more personal. What happens when the strain on the healthcare system results in longer wait times, reduced access to specialists, or decreased funding for preventative programs? The people who suffer the most are often those who have the least power to change their circumstances. Low-income families, the elderly, and children are disproportionately impacted by the diversion of resources. Smoking, in many ways, preys on the vulnerable, and the financial strain it creates only deepens that inequity.

Let's take a moment to reflect on this. I will use the dollar as an example here, but the same example works for any denomination. For every dollar spent treating smoking-related illnesses, there's a cost that isn't measured in numbers. It's measured in the lives of people who go untreated for other conditions because the resources simply aren't there. It's measured in the reduced quality of care for patients who did nothing to invite this crisis into their lives. It's measured in the growing sense of frustration, helplessness, and anger among those who see their healthcare system failing to meet their needs because it's too busy dealing with a preventable problem.

We've been conditioned to think of smoking as a personal choice, a matter of individual freedom. But when that choice puts an entire healthcare system under pressure, it stops being just about the individual. It becomes a matter of public responsibility. And we have to stop pretending otherwise.

As we explore the financial burden of smoking, it's important to recognize that these costs aren't just abstract figures. They represent a failure of priorities, a willingness to allow preventable harm to continue at the expense of public health. And the consequences aren't just felt in hospitals and government budgets. They're felt in the everyday lives of people who pay higher premiums, face longer wait times, and experience reduced access to quality care.

Imagine that every year, your country, or every single country in this world for that matter, would load a truck with BILLIONS in denomination. Drive to a pit of fire, back up the truck and unload all that money into the pit, burning it, while everyone watches and think it is the most acceptable thing there is. There is no benefit to smoking and there isn't one justifiable reason to spend any amount of time or money defending it.

So, what do we do about it? The solution isn't just about shifting blame or pointing fingers. It's about shifting the narrative. It's about recognizing that smoking is more than just a habit, it's a societal issue that requires collective action. This isn't a battle that can be fought with isolated regulations or half-hearted campaigns. It requires a commitment to changing the culture, shifting public perception, and demanding accountability from the industries that profit from our collective suffering.

The bottom line is this: The financial fallout from smoking is more than just a line item on a balance sheet. It's a reflection of a broken system, a system that prioritizes individual profit over collective well-being, and short-term convenience over long-term health. And it's up to all of us to demand better.

If you've made it this far, you're already part of the solution. You're willing to confront the uncomfortable truth and acknowledge the bigger picture. And that's the first step. Because the road to change starts with awareness, and awareness starts with seeing smoking for what it really is, not just a personal habit, but a public health crisis that impacts all of us, smoking leads to the ultimate destination in the *Cancer Highway*: strain, suffering and death. The financial burden isn't just about dollars and cents; it's about lives, priorities, and the choices we make as a society. Let's start making better ones.

Emotional Impact

It's easy to conceptualise the scope of the financial costs of smoking to an extent, the hospital bills, the medical expenses, the lost productivity, and think that's where the impact ends. But there's another side to this, one that can't be quantified on a spreadsheet or accounted for in a budget. This is the emotional toll, the way smoking fractures friendships, weighs down families, and leaves a trail of grief and frustration in its wake. It's a price that every smoker and non-smoker pay, in one way or another, and it's often invisible until it hits home.

We don't often think about the way smoking can put a strain on friendships, but it happens more than you'd expect. Picture this: you're a non-smoker and you're out with a close friend, someone you care about deeply, and you're enjoying a conversation when they light up a cigarette. Maybe you're used to it by now; maybe you're not. But either way, there's an unspoken tension that arises. It's not just about the discomfort of breathing in smoke. It's the silent wedge it drives between you, a barrier made of toxins and health risks that neither of you fully acknowledges.

For many non-smokers, it's not just an irritation; it's a genuine source of stress and concern. Watching someone you care about willingly put their health at risk is difficult enough. But being forced to share in that risk, to breathe in the second-hand smoke and face the consequences of their choice, is something else entirely. Over time, this tension can erode the foundation of a friendship. It creates an environment where conversations are laced with silent judgments and concerns that never quite make it to the surface.

How many times have you stood awkwardly by as a friend takes a smoke break, feeling torn between your desire to stay connected and your discomfort with the situation? Or perhaps you've found yourself avoiding certain gatherings or activities because you know they'll be filled with cigarette smoke. These are also hidden costs of smoking, the quiet sacrifices and compromises that non-smokers make to maintain relationships, often at the expense of their own health and well-being.

Look at it from the point of view of a smoker, at least those conscious enough of the damages of their choice of habit. Imagine you are a smoker, knowing all there is to know about the habit, and wherever you go you will light up your cigarette, you are aware that your toxic smoke is travelling somewhere, over onto someone, to a passer-by or even your friends who are gathering nearby or next to you, that every breath they take is causing them harm and it is all because your habit. You are forcing people to be the passengers on this journey across the *Cancer Highway*, against their will, and there is no way that you can travel that road without taking unwilling people with you.

And then, there are the families left behind, bearing the brunt of the emotional and financial fallout from smoking-related deaths. Losing a loved one to a smoking-related illness is a pain that lingers long after the funeral. It's not just the physical absence that hurts, but the knowledge that the loss could have been prevented. For many, this grief is compounded by a sense of helplessness and anger. Anger at the tobacco industry for its relentless fight to keep the toxic habit discreet and prevalent. Anger at the lack of awareness and accountability. And sometimes, anger at the smoker themselves for the choices that led to this outcome.

When someone dies from a smoking-related illness, it's not just their life that ends. It's the countless moments they'll never get to share with their family, the graduations, the weddings, the quiet Sunday mornings. For every smoker who loses their life, there are children left without a parent, spouses left without a partner, and friends left with a void that can never be filled. And in many cases, these victims weren't even the ones holding the cigarette. They were the innocent bystanders; the unwilling passengers' smokers took on that ride.

The harsh reality is that many of the victims of smoking are non-smokers who were exposed through no fault of their own. These are the children growing up in smoke-filled homes, developing respiratory issues and chronic illnesses that will follow them for the rest of their lives. These are the spouses who watch their partners suffer through long, painful battles with lung cancer or heart disease, all the while knowing that it could have been avoided.

And then there are the parents who have to bury their children, victims of second-hand smoke or smoking-related complications. Imagine the guilt and heartbreak of losing a child to something so preventable, knowing that their suffering was the result of someone else's habit. It's a weight that no parent should have to bear, and yet it happens far too often.

Globally, around 40% of children are regularly exposed to second-hand smoke at home. According to data from organizations such as the World Health Organization (WHO) and UNICEF, the harm caused by second-hand smoke in children is substantial. Each year, an estimated 65,000 to 70,000 children die due to infections related to second-hand smoke, such as pneumonia, bronchitis, and other acute respiratory conditions. When it comes to pre-natal exposures, 166,000 annual infant deaths are attributed to complications from maternal smoking, including low birth weight, preterm birth, and SIDS.

It's not just the immediate exposure to cigarette smoke that causes harm. Let me repeat myself here a little bit. As I spoke in chapter 2, even after the cigarette is extinguished, the toxins linger in the air, on clothing, and in the very walls of a home, the insidious third-hand smoke, and it poses a silent threat to anyone who lives in or visits a smoker's home. For families with children, this can be especially dangerous. Studies have shown that third-hand smoke can persist in homes for months after a smoker quits, exposing children to harmful chemicals long after the last cigarette is put out.

For non-smokers who live with or regularly visit smokers, this lingering presence of third-hand smoke can create a constant sense of unease. It's a reminder that, no matter how careful a smoker tries to be, the consequences of their habit extend far beyond their own body. It's a source of frustration and helplessness, knowing that you're breathing in toxins every time you enter a room, despite having no say in the matter.

Living with a chronic illness caused by second-hand smoke is not just a physical burden; it's an overwhelmingly emotional one. For many non-smokers, the realization that their health issues are the result of someone else's habit can be infuriating. It's a constant reminder that their suffering could have been avoided if only the people around them had made different choices. This sense of injustice can weigh heavily on a person's mental health, leading to feelings of resentment, anger, and even depression.

Imagine being diagnosed with a chronic respiratory illness, knowing that you never chose to smoke a cigarette in your life. You did everything right, avoided smoking, stayed healthy, made good choices, and yet, here you are, living with the consequences of someone else's actions. It's a bitter pill to swallow, and it's one that far too many non-smokers are forced to take.

In social situations, the presence of smoking can create an invisible divide between smokers and non-smokers. There's the unspoken understanding that, at some point, the smokers will step outside for a cigarette, leaving the non-smokers behind. For non-smokers, this can create a sense of exclusion and discomfort, as if they're being left out of the conversation simply because they choose not to smoke. It's a small thing, but over time, these moments of exclusion can add up, creating a rift that slowly pushes people apart. I'm often victim of this one specifically, I am often ostracised for being the one who stands up against being that victim, I will not hang around my good friends who smokes and I'm the one seen as the unreasonable one.

Even when the group gather again, the lingering smell of smoke can serve as a reminder of the divide. It's not just an unpleasant odour; it's a symbol of the differing choices and priorities that separate smokers from non-smokers. And for those who are particularly sensitive to cigarette smoke, this can be a source of ongoing stress and irritation, making social interactions feel like a minefield of potential triggers.

Don't even let me get started on kissing a smoker, if you are a smoker and wants to know what your breath smells like, take a used ashtray still full of ashes and cigarette butts, pour hot water on it and breathe it in, that is what a smokers breath smells like and the kiss tastes like.

The emotional impact of smoking goes beyond the individual smoker. It affects friendships, families, and entire communities. It's the strain of watching someone you care about make choices that put their health at risk. It's the frustration of being exposed to second-hand smoke, despite your best efforts to avoid it. And it's the grief of losing a loved one to a preventable illness, knowing that their death didn't have to happen.

It's time we start recognizing these hidden costs and acknowledging the emotional toll that smoking takes on non-smokers. Because at the end of the day, smoking is a choice that impacts everyone around you. And those impacts aren't just financial, they're deeply personal, affecting the way we connect with each other and navigate our relationships.

If we're going to address the smoking crisis, we need to do more than just count the monetary loss and the lives shortened. We need to understand the full scope of the damage, from the strained friendships and fractured families to the lingering grief and quiet resentment. Only then can we truly grasp the cost of smoking, and only then can we begin to demand change.

Part 2: The Psychology of Addiction and the Glorification of Smoking

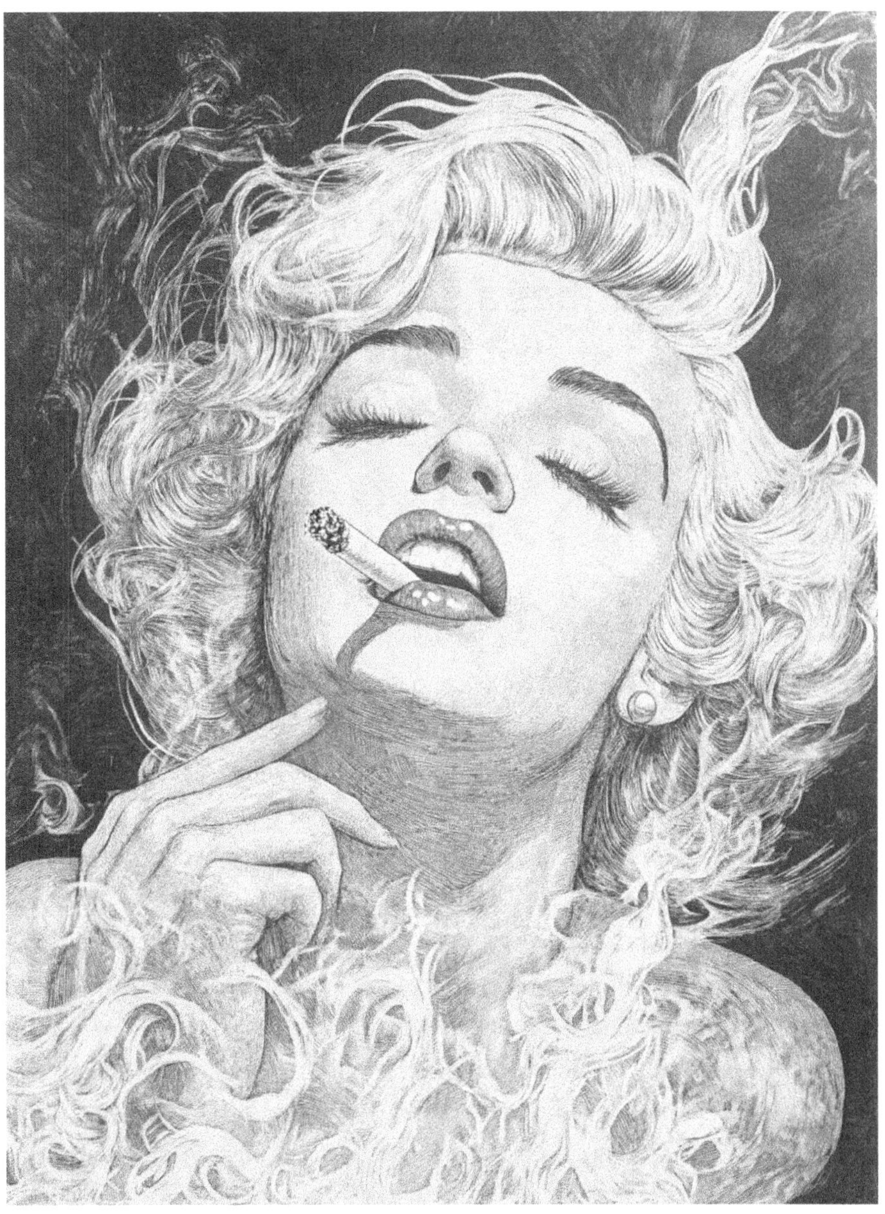

Chapter 4 | The Cool Killer – How Society Glorifies a Deadly Habit

hink back to the last movie you watched. Maybe the lead character was a hardened detective with a cigarette dangling from their lips, or a rockstar framed in shadows, exhaling smoke as if it were a part of their untamed, iconic spirit. Or perhaps it was a social media influencer, casually holding a vape pen like the latest coveted accessory. These images carry a powerful punch, not because they demand attention, but because they slip in subtly, connecting a deadly habit to people society has elevated, even idolized. We see their defiant edge, their allure, and unconsciously absorb the message: if they're doing it, it must be worth the risk.

It's not just about falling victim of smoking habits; it's about the way society glorifies certain people and how that status grants them an undeniable influence over the rest of us. When someone we admire picks up a cigarette, it's rarely questioned, it becomes just another part of their charm, their mystique. This sway is quiet, almost unnoticeable, yet potent. What happens, though, when the habits they embody are harmful? What does it say about us, about our culture, that a behaviour capable of shortening lives and devastating health can ride along on the coattails of someone's glamour, getting a pass simply because it's wrapped in prestige?

You've heard of the phrase "Monkey See Monkey Do". In this chapter I want to dive into this complex territory where culture, media, and health collide: how has society managed to glorify a habit that kills simply by becoming more susceptive to and even mimicking figures we admire? And what does it reveal about the subtle yet impactful messages we absorb every day?

Media Representation

When we think about movies and TV shows, it's not just what's said that leaves an impression, it's what's shown, what's repeated, and what's glamorized. And when it comes to smoking, the portrayal is nothing short of a masterclass in deception. Through a polished lens, the media has managed to turn an act that is essentially self-harm into a mark of allure, mystery, and rebellion. Think about it: How many times have you seen the "cool" character casually lighting up, staring off into the distance as if they hold all the secrets of the universe? It's everywhere, like an invisible but persistent whisper that says, "This is what being cool looks like." And therein lies the danger.

Movies and television often present smoking as an aesthetic, a part of a character's identity, or an expression of defiance. Characters like James Dean in *Rebel Without a Cause* or a more modern example like Uma Thurman in *Pulp Fiction* are etched into our memories, cigarettes hanging loosely between their fingers. It's not just a prop; it's a signal to the audience, this person is edgy, interesting, and complex. That cigarette isn't just a cigarette, it's a metaphor for confidence, nonchalance, or even tragedy. The problem is that these associations blur the lines between fiction and reality, leaving young and impressionable minds to pick up more than just storylines.

In many ways, the screen has been a more effective salesman than the tobacco industry ever was. Between the 1930s and 1950s, when Hollywood was in its Golden Age, smoking became synonymous with sophistication and charm. Actors like Humphrey Bogart and actresses like Audrey Hepburn weren't just stars, they were icons. And with every puff they took, they transformed smoking into an aspirational act, something desirable to emulate. But even today, decades after the link between smoking and deadly diseases has been made undeniably clear, the legacy of that era lingers on.

One study published in *The Lancet* highlighted that, young adults who see smoking portrayed as glamorous or rebellious in movies are twice as likely to take up the habit themselves. This isn't just a statistic; it's a reflection of human behaviour. We're wired to imitate, to want to belong, and when smoking is continually shown as a sign of independence or sophistication, the seeds are sown for real-world consequences. It's not by chance that smoking among teens surged in the mid-90s with the rise of grunge culture and movies like *Trainspotting*, where smoking and drug use were portrayed not just as vices, but as elements of authenticity.

What's more, we rarely see the consequences of this behaviour on-screen. The hacking coughs, the gradual deterioration of lung tissue, the slow decay of vitality, these real-life horrors are noticeably absent. In a world that glamorizes cigarette breaks, where are the images of oxygen tanks, tracheotomies, and last goodbyes at hospital bedsides? It's a sanitized version of reality that keeps the audience entertained, while the truth smoulders in the background. This selective storytelling is more than misleading; it's manipulative.

For all the information we know about smoking, you'd think media platforms would carry more responsibility. After all, if a soda company is required to mention the sugar content on its label, shouldn't a movie glorifying cigarettes come with a health warning? But that's not what we see. Hollywood and mainstream media continue to serve up smoking scenes without a hint of caution, normalizing an addictive and deadly habit. And let's be real, it's more than just negligence. It's irresponsible.

To add some perspective, a movie that shows self-harm will be forced to put a disclaimer somewhere. Smoking is self-harm, but it doesn't limit itself to the user, it causes harm to those around the smokers and even indirectly linked to them. Just because it happens at a lower pace, it doesn't mean it is any less important to acknowledge.

Imagine watching a movie where the lead character is shown consuming dangerous amounts of alcohol without ever facing any consequences. After a while, you start to believe that this behaviour is just a part of life, without realizing you're absorbing a narrative that can potentially harm you. The same applies to smoking scenes. It's the repetition, the glamorization, and the lack of visible consequences that engrain the behaviour into our collective consciousness.

Today's battlefield has shifted from the big screen to smaller screens that fit into the palm of our hands. Social media influencers and celebrities are the new idols, and their actions carry immense weight. Even as smoking has declined in public spaces, the idea of a cigarette as an accessory to a certain "aesthetic" persists. Look at how many Instagram posts or YouTube vlogs depict vaping in stylish, curated snapshots. The carefully crafted images of e-cigarettes paired with high fashion, urban streetwear, or a moody, contemplative look send the message loud and clear: smoking isn't just a habit, it's an identity.

I will cover more about the vaping habit and how it recently is strongly associated with being the gateway to learn to smoke to a lot of people. While no specific celebrity or influencer is well known to publicly depict vaping and smoking as a desirable habit, many of them will low-key glamorise it to their audience, framing the device and the smoke patterns as stylish.

Yet again, we find ourselves in a situation where the appeal is enhanced, but the cost is left unspoken. What's missing from these photos and videos is the image of someone struggling for breath after a few flights of stairs, or the look on a doctor's face delivering the worst kind of news. It's like watching someone cruise down the *Cancer Highway*, blissfully unaware that they're speeding straight towards the end.

So why is this a big deal? Why does it matter if media and social media keep glorifying smoking? Because, at its core, smoking is still a leading cause of preventable death worldwide. The World Health Organization estimates that smoking kills over 8 million people every year. And the reality is, not all smokers make a conscious decision to start. Many are influenced by these glamorized images and subtle suggestions that smoking is the key to being interesting or rebellious. But once hooked, they find themselves on a highway to cancer and heart disease with no exit in sight.

The goal here isn't to demonize every movie that's ever shown a character smoking. It's to shine a light on the impact these portrayals have on people who don't yet have the life experience to separate fiction from reality. Imagine a young adult watching their favourite actor light up, looking impossibly cool, or their favourite influencer doing the same. That teenager doesn't see the actor sitting down with a director, discussing lighting and camera angles. They don't see the crew planning the shot to make it visually appealing, similar approach for the influencer who is trying to capture the best shot. All they see is a role model doing something intriguing, and that image stays with them long after.

It's time to stop pretending these portrayals are harmless. They're not just scenes on the screen, they're messages, repeated often enough to become beliefs. Smoking is more than a plot device or a visual cue, it's a real, life-altering addiction with a death toll that doesn't lie. We owe it to future generations to challenge the media's romanticized version of this deadly habit and start telling the truth, even if it isn't as glamorous.

The Danger of Nostalgia

Nostalgia is a powerful thing. It has this almost magical way of warping time, wrapping our memories in a hazy glow that softens the rough edges of the past. It's why we romanticize certain eras, why the 1950s feels like a golden age of glamour, or why we cling to images of Old Hollywood and its starlets. But there's a darker side to nostalgia, and it's not as harmless as it seems. One of the most insidious aspects of looking back through rose-tinted glasses is how easily it can mask the dangers that were once normalized, like smoking.

Think of the iconic black-and-white images of classic movie stars. There's Audrey Hepburn in *Breakfast at Tiffany's*, with her cigarette holder gracefully extended, embodying elegance and sophistication. Or James Dean, leaning against a car, cigarette in hand, gazing broodingly into the distance. These images are more than just snapshots of a bygone era; they've become cultural artifacts that represent something larger. They symbolize style, rebellion, and allure. They evoke a sense of longing for a time when everything seemed simpler, or maybe just better.

But nostalgia doesn't tell the whole story. The truth is that these images, which have been immortalized in pop culture, carry with them an implied message: smoking is part of what made these people iconic. It's as if the cigarette was a key to their mystique, an accessory that added to their appeal. And when we view these images through a nostalgic lens, we forget that these portrayals were not only culturally significant, they were also harmful. They were marketing tools for an industry that thrived on creating addicts, shaping public perception to turn smoking into a rite of passage.

Nostalgia plays tricks on us. It takes the harsh reality of smoking and edits it out of the frame, leaving us with a polished fantasy. And it's not just the distant past. Consider how the resurgence of vintage styles keeps bringing back elements of past decades, from retro fashion to mid-century modern furniture. Inevitably, smoking comes along for the ride. It's as if when we try to recapture a time period, we unintentionally resurrect its mistakes as well.

This is where the danger lies, especially for young people who are drawn to these nostalgic trends. When someone today looks back at old Hollywood or flips through a magazine featuring photos of musicians in the 70s, what they see is an aesthetic. A mood. A vibe. They see the cigarette, but not the context. They don't see the rise in lung cancer rates that followed Hollywood's peak or the fact that many of these stars didn't live long enough to enjoy their legendary status.

Imagine this: A teenager fascinated by the glamour of the past starts curating their social media feed with black-and-white photos of classic Hollywood stars. They find images of Marilyn Monroe lounging, cigarette in hand, or Bob Dylan performing with a lit cigarette perched on his guitar. As they scroll, they absorb these visuals without realizing that this "timeless cool" they're idolizing was often built on a deadly habit. Nostalgia seduces with the appeal of yesteryear's charm but keeps its deadly consequences just out of frame.

In the same way, the 1950s and 60s are often painted as a time of unmatched glamour, sophistication, and style. But beneath that shiny exterior was a world where smoking was pervasive. The images that persist from those eras reinforce a myth: that smoking was just part of the ambiance, an almost required accessory for anyone who wanted to be taken seriously or seen as stylish. It's hard to ignore the enduring allure of these images, even for those who understand the harm smoking causes.

If you've ever watched old cartoons, you might have noticed that some now come with disclaimers, warnings that acknowledge and condemn the racial stereotypes they contain. It's a progressive step, acknowledging the wrongs of the past instead of erasing them. Warner Bros. knew that it was the right thing to do, to say to today's audiences, "Yes, this happened, and it wasn't okay." But why do we still fall short when it comes to harmful habits like smoking? Where are the warnings on classic films, television shows, or even old advertisements that made smoking look essential to being sophisticated, rebellious, or powerful?

Imagine a similar disclaimer before an old black-and-white movie: "Smoking is a deadly and addictive habit that was once glamorized but is now known to cause cancer and numerous other diseases." It's a small step, but it shifts the lens just enough to change how the audience interprets what they see. It's acknowledging that while this portrayal may have been normal in the past, we now know better. And when you know better, you have a responsibility to do better.

This cultural nostalgia isn't confined to just the big screen. We see it in the modern-day revival of jazz bars, vintage fashion trends, and even the resurgence of vinyl records. It's a longing for something "authentic" or "raw" that's driven these trends, and it's no accident that smoking fits neatly into this picture. There's a reason people still use the term "smoke-filled jazz club" to conjure a sense of moody sophistication. But when we romanticize these scenes, we don't often think about the long-term health impacts of inhaling that smoke, whether you're holding the cigarette or just sitting in the room.

The term *Cancer Highway* isn't an exaggeration here. Smoking laid the path, paved it with seductive imagery and a promise of something more, a more exciting life, a deeper personality, a clearer identity. But as we've learned from the staggering numbers of people who have suffered due to tobacco, this road only leads one way. And nostalgia, with all its charm, often puts blinders on our understanding of that reality.

For many of today's youth, smoking seems like a relic of the past, a throwback to their grandparents' time or old black-and-white films. And yet, vintage culture thrives among younger generations. They seek out what's old, what's classic, what's retro. But how do they separate the appeal of the aesthetic from the danger of its normalized habits?

That's where we, as a society, need to step in and fill the gaps that nostalgia leaves behind. We need to acknowledge that while the past had its allure, it also had its pitfalls. It's not about demonizing the stars or condemning the art. It's about being honest. James Dean may have been the icon of youthful rebellion, but let's not forget that he was also part of an industry that helped market a product designed to addict and kill. Audrey Hepburn may have embodied grace and elegance, but we can still admire her without promoting the unhealthy habits that were once so normalized.

This isn't an attack on the past. It's a reminder that we have to learn from it. Nostalgia can be beautiful, but it can also be deceptive. We need to find a balance between appreciating what was and acknowledging what wasn't okay. Because if we don't, we risk creating a whole new generation of people who look back and only see the beauty, not the danger.

It's time to put the rose-tinted glasses aside and see nostalgia for what it is: a mixed bag of cultural memories, some of which should stay in the past. It's time to break the connection between vintage charm and smoking's dark legacy. Romanticizing the past doesn't mean ignoring the mistakes that were made, it means recognizing them and being clear about the lessons we've learned. And one of the most critical lessons is this: Smoking isn't stylish, glamorous, or cool. It never was.

The Social Media Glorification of the Unhealthy "Cool"

If you ever doubt the influence of social media, look around next time you're out. Look at children and teenagers scrolling through their phones, absorbing images that shape their ideas of what's trendy, what's stylish, and what's "cool." And look even closer, have you ever personally seen a child vaping?

Or watched as a teen blows a cloud of vapor for the camera, capturing it all in slow motion to post online? This isn't a rare sight anymore. In fact, it's become a new normal, and it's no accident.

In today's world, the idea of "cool" isn't just something whispered through the walls of high school cafeterias or discussed in the lyrics of popular songs. It's a powerful, ever-present undercurrent that flows through every like, every share, and every post. The most dangerous thing about this current is that it's unfiltered and fast-moving. Social media isn't just changing what's trending, it's reshaping how young people perceive habits, lifestyles, and risks. What's seen as aspirational, sexy, or rebellious is now curated on a feed, and smoking, in its new avatar of vaping, is once again at the heart of this twisted portrayal.

What once took years of cinema to instil, social media can accomplish in days. Platforms like Instagram, TikTok, and Snapchat are the new Hollywood, and the reach is far more personal and intimate. Young people idolize influencers in ways that surpass the reverence held for movie stars of previous generations. And these influencers? They aren't selling you a movie ticket; they're selling you a lifestyle, an image, an identity.

Think about the way smoking is replaced with vaping, a sleek, modern evolution of the cigarette that promises the same allure without the unpleasant smell. The devices are marketed in an array of colours and designs, making them more like stylish accessories than harmful products. Now, mix in social media influencers who casually showcase their vaping in glamorous shots, dramatic videos, or in laid-back settings that suggest relaxation and rebellion. What we're witnessing is the rebranding of smoking, disguised as something edgy and sophisticated.

It's not that different from the old movies we discussed previously, where smoking was made to look like an essential part of being mysterious, so-phisticated, or dangerous. The difference today is that the medium isn't passive. Social media invites interaction, demands engagement, and thrives on imitation. The images are curated, but the consequences are real.

Let's talk about influencers for a moment. On social media, these individuals have become the new architects of culture. They set trends, shape perceptions, and hold more sway over a young audience than any advertising campaign could dream of. And the tobacco industry knows it. Take JUUL, for example. The e-cigarette giant was caught red-handed in an orchestrated effort to appeal to younger audiences through social media influencers, online campaigns, and flashy events. It wasn't an oversight; it was a strategy. A strategy that preyed on the vulnerable, capitalizing on the aspirational nature of social media to lure in kids and teens.

These influencers didn't explicitly tell their young followers to start vaping. They didn't need to. By simply integrating vaping into their curated lives, set against the backdrop of concerts, fashion shows, road trips, and weekend getaways, they sent a clear message: This is what's cool. This is what the in-crowd is doing. If you want to belong, you should try it too. And the numbers prove it.

In the USA, according to a study from the National Institute on Drug Abuse, the percentage of high school seniors who reported vaping nicotine jumped from 11% in 2017 to nearly 25% in 2019. That's not a small jump, it's a tidal wave. One that swept millions of young people onto a path they might not have taken otherwise. The allure of being "cool" on social media, combined with the normalization of vaping, is driving these teens down a road paved with nicotine addiction and health risks that we're only beginning to fully understand.

Here's the kicker: Vaping isn't as safe as the sleek ads and influencer posts would have you believe. According to a report by the CDC, nearly 3 million middle and high school students in the United States admitted to vaping in 2021. And while the short-term effects might seem negligible, head rushes, quick buzzes, the long-term consequences are stacking up. Vaping-related lung illnesses have already claimed lives and hospitalized thousands.

And yet, this threat remains largely under the radar because it's disguised as something trendy. It's promoted with hashtags, slow-motion effects, and filters that make it seem like just another part of a modern lifestyle. But in reality, these kids are getting hooked on nicotine, one of the most addictive substances ON THE PLANET, and heading down the same *Cancer Highway* we've seen before. It's just paved with sleeker, shinier billboards this time around.

The real tragedy here is that many young people believe they're making a healthier choice. That's the narrative they've been sold. They've been told that vaping is a safer alternative to smoking. And while it's true that vaping cuts out some of the toxic chemicals found in traditional cigarettes, it's far from harmless. It's like being told you're taking a shortcut, only to find out that it leads you straight off a cliff. To an addicted, switching to cigarettes becomes a logical next step, especially as tolerance builds and vaping alone fails to provide the same rush. The initial choice to vape often sets in motion a chain reaction that can drag users down the *Cancer Highway*, from sleek vape pens to deadly tobacco

Part of this "healthier alternative" misconception comes from a lack of visible consequences. When you see a celebrity or an influencer vaping, you don't see them coughing up tar, dealing with reduced lung capacity, or struggling with chronic bronchitis. Just like old Hollywood masked the real consequences of smoking, social media hides the very real dangers of vaping.

So, where do we go from here? How do we break this cycle of glorifying an unhealthy "cool" that's so deeply embedded in the digital age? We start by acknowledging the power that social media wields and holding it accountable. Platforms like Instagram and TikTok aren't just windows into someone's life; they're powerful tools of influence that can shape real-world behaviour. And just as we've seen disclaimers added to old movies warning about outdated stereotypes, we need these platforms to step up and address the glorification of smoking and vaping.

It's not enough to ban ads from the tobacco industry. These companies are savvy, and they've already adapted by partnering with influencers who aren't under the same scrutiny. There's a reason you don't see warnings at the beginning of an influencer's video, even if that video casually features vaping. But these disclaimers aren't just about pointing fingers, they're about giving viewers context, about educating the next generation so they can recognize the illusion for what it is.

Ultimately, it's up to us, as a society, to guide younger generations through this minefield. We need to teach them to look beyond the filters, beyond the likes, and understand the full picture. Smoking, in all its forms, isn't cool, sophisticated, or glamorous, it's a slow and relentless path to addiction and disease. And those who promote it, knowingly or unknowingly, are pushing others towards that path without showing them where it leads.

Social media might be an essential part of life now, but that doesn't mean we can't control the messages it sends. We need to unmask the dangers hiding behind the likes, behind the curated lifestyles, and show that what's marketed as cool today can cost a lifetime of health tomorrow. And for those who are already struggling with nicotine addiction, we owe them empathy, support, and encouragement, not judgment. The struggle is real, but so are the stakes. The road ahead might be tempting, but we have to make sure they know what's waiting at the end of it.

Chapter 5 | Peer Pressure and Social Smoking – Why People Still Start

Social pressure is a quiet yet potent force that shapes our choices, often in ways we barely notice. At its core, social pressure taps into a basic human need for belonging; we are wired to seek connection and avoid isolation. This instinct makes us highly sensitive to the cues of those around us, leading us to conform to group norms, even if it goes against our better judgment. In trying to fit in, we often find ourselves more willing to make small compromises that, over time, can add up to much larger shifts in behaviour or values.

One of the ways social pressure makes us vulnerable is by encouraging us to prioritize acceptance over authenticity. When we face a decision in a group setting, whether it's smoking at a party, engaging in risky behaviour, or simply going along with an opinion we don't fully agree with, the fear of exclusion often outweighs our individual preferences. This subtle influence can blur the line between what we genuinely want and what we think we *should* want in order to belong.

This vulnerability is especially impactful because it happens gradually, without overt coercion. Small actions taken "just to fit in" can lead to habits or behaviours that don't reflect our true selves. Recognizing the power of social pressure allows us to make choices more consciously, embracing our own values and boundaries rather than yielding to the silent, pervasive tug of conformity.

The Social Pull

Imagine a crowded party, lights dim, laughter spilling from every corner, music vibrating through the room. Just outside, illuminated by the faint glow of garden lights, a group huddles together. A hand passes a cigarette to the next person, who takes a drag, then another. It's a simple scene but look closer, something powerful is happening here. It's not just about smoking. It's about connection, about the subtle promise of inclusion that smoking seems to hold. In that moment, holding a cigarette doesn't feel like a health risk. It feels like a ticket to belonging, a way of saying, *I'm part of this.* To someone, that will be their first time in that circle, to someone that will be their first time being passed a cigarette and the fear of standing out will likely shape their next decision in anchoring them in this brief moment of camaraderie.

This is how the grip of social smoking starts. The lure is not the smoke itself but the sense of companionship it appears to bring. Research shows that humans are wired to seek connection, to belong, and to avoid standing out in a way that might lead to rejection. Social smoking taps into this need with precision. It turns a dangerous habit into a bonding ritual, making it not just easy to start but hard to resist. The pressure is rarely overt; no one is forcing that cigarette into anyone's hand. But the pull is undeniable, especially for young people stepping into new social landscapes, trying to navigate a world that often feels as uncertain as it is exciting.

The act of smoking in these moments can feel like a natural part of social life, especially in environments like parties, bars, and break rooms where people gather, laugh, and share stories. A cigarette becomes more than tobacco and paper; it's a symbol, a gesture, a bridge that connects strangers and friends alike. But beneath this casual exchange lies a darker reality. For many, social smoking becomes the first step onto a path that can lead to a lifelong addiction, a dangerous highway which path leads to a precipice. And this path doesn't just affect the smoker. Each puff affects the air around them, subtly impacting the health of everyone nearby. The hidden cost that no one thinks about in that warm, easy glow of social connection.

Statistics illustrate just how influential this pull can be. Studies reveal that nearly 70% of smokers began in social settings, often around friends or acquaintances who smoked. It's not surprising. When everyone around you is smoking, refusing can feel like stepping away from the group itself. For a young person at a bar, surrounded by friends who all have cigarettes in hand, choosing to stay cigarette-free feels like a choice to stand apart, to risk feeling like an outsider. And that's a powerful deterrent because, as humans, we're wired to avoid rejection. Even when we know the risks intellectually, the emotional pull of belonging often wins out.

Social smoking also brings a troubling sense of denial. Many people consider themselves "only social smokers" as though this distinction grants immunity from the harms of tobacco. They convince themselves it's harmless because they only smoke occasionally, at gatherings or celebrations. But every "social" cigarette is still a cigarette, filled with the same toxic chemicals, carrying the same risks of addiction and disease. This belief, that social smoking is somehow safer or less serious, creates a false sense of security that blinds people to the danger they're stepping into. It's like dipping your toe into quicksand and believing you won't sink because you're only "sort of" in it.

The social pull of smoking is perhaps strongest during moments of transition, especially for young people. Entering college, moving to a new city, or starting a new job, all of these changes create a heightened need for connection, making the pull of social smoking even stronger. In these moments, a cigarette can feel like a small price to pay for a sense of belonging. Young people especially are vulnerable to this pull; the desire to fit in is at its peak, and social smoking becomes an easy way to bridge that gap. What starts as a casual gesture can evolve into a dependency before they even realize it. Studies on adolescent smoking show that those who begin smoking socially are far more likely to become regular smokers than those who never picked up a cigarette in social settings.

But the truth is, this "small price" is anything but. Social smoking can spiral into full addiction over time, not because it's an intense craving from the start but because it becomes familiar. With each social cigarette, the body becomes accustomed to nicotine, creating a growing tolerance and increasing dependence. And by the time someone realizes they're smoking more often than they intended, they're already far down that path, moving from the occasional "social" cigarette to a regular habit.

The social aspect doesn't just encourage people to start smoking; it also makes it difficult to stop. Picture a smoker trying to quit. They go to a party, and everyone around them is lighting up, offering them a cigarette, laughing, talking. The sense of temptation is heightened by that same sense of belonging, making it harder to say no and stay on the quitting path. In this way, social settings don't just encourage smoking; they reinforce it, pulling those trying to quit back into the habit, trapping them in a cycle that's difficult to break.

When we talk about smoking, we often focus on its health risks, lung cancer, heart disease, respiratory issues. And those are all real, deadly consequences. But we also have to acknowledge the social forces at play, the way peer dynamics make smoking seem almost inevitable in certain situations. And it's here that the cycle of social smoking thrives, passing from one generation to the next. Because as long as smoking is framed as a social norm, an "acceptable" way to bond, we'll continue to see people, especially young people, lured down this path.

So, what can we do? The first step is awareness, understanding that social pressure is not just harmless fun. It's a powerful force that exploits our need to belong. Recognizing this is key to breaking the cycle, to making choices rooted in genuine connection rather than the need for approval. When we see social smoking for what it truly is, a dangerous detour disguised as a social bridge, we gain the power to step away, to say no, and to redefine what connection really means.

The social pull of smoking may be strong, but it's not unbeatable. By recognizing the underlying influences, by challenging the belief that smoking is just a harmless part of social life, we can start to shift the narrative. We can create spaces where people don't have to choose between health and belonging, where connection is built on authenticity, not addiction. It starts with awareness, with one choice at a time, each choice breaking the hold of this social pull, leading us towards a culture where health and connection go hand in hand.

The Myth of Occasional Smoking

There's no safe version of smoking. Yet the myth of occasional smoking has convinced millions otherwise. It's a belief that has quietly embedded itself into social consciousness, whispering a comforting, dangerous lie, that smoking in moderation, "just once in a while," or "I only smoke when I drink", somehow protects you from the risks of addiction and health damage. But this idea couldn't be further from the truth. Occasional smoking may seem like a harmless habit, but it's a slippery, deceptive path, one that invites all the same risks and dangers as regular smoking, just dressed in subtler clothes.

The brain's response to nicotine plays a central role in keeping this myth alive. With every cigarette, even one smoked occasionally, nicotine enters the bloodstream, travels to the brain, and releases a surge of dopamine, a neurotransmitter responsible for pleasure and reward. This dopamine "hit" is what keeps smokers coming back, often without them even realizing it. Nicotine hijacks the brain's reward system, which has evolved to reinforce behaviours necessary for survival, like eating or social bonding. But nicotine hacks into that system, tricking the brain into treating smoking as something rewarding, something worth repeating.

And here's where the myth of occasional smoking takes root: the brain doesn't distinguish between an occasional reward and a regular one. Neurologically, each cigarette strengthens neural pathways, building a habit loop. Even with intermittent smoking, these dopamine hits prime the brain to associate cigarettes with satisfaction and pleasure. Over time, this association deepens, and even the occasional smoker finds themselves with a growing urge for more. Each cigarette, whether it's once a day or once a month, strengthens this craving, reinforcing the pathway that links nicotine to pleasure, making future cravings harder to ignore.

In fact, studies show that nicotine's addictive grip can take hold remarkably quickly, with even occasional smokers reporting withdrawal symptoms when they try to cut back. The American Heart Association notes that nicotine is one of the most addictive substances available, ranking alongside drugs like heroin and cocaine. And like these substances, nicotine reprograms the brain, leaving even infrequent users with psychological and physiological dependencies that make it difficult to resist the next cigarette.

The power of nicotine dependency lies not just in its physical effects but in its ability to create mental habits that latch onto social behaviours. This is where the myth of occasional smoking becomes especially dangerous. Social settings become "cues" for smoking, where the brain starts associating parties, gatherings, or certain people with the rewarding experience of a cigarette. It creates an environment where occasional smokers don't feel addicted because they only smoke under specific conditions. However, these very conditions serve as psychological triggers, reinforcing cravings each time they're in a similar setting. This conditioning forms a cycle that can pull occasional smokers closer to regular smoking patterns without them even noticing.

The myth of occasional smoking is further sustained by our brains' tendency to rationalize and justify behaviours. In psychology, this phenomenon is known as "cognitive dissonance", the discomfort we feel when our actions don't align with our beliefs. Occasional smokers know that smoking is harmful, yet they continue. To resolve this dissonance, the brain subtly shifts its narrative, telling itself that occasional smoking is different, safer, or even insignificant compared to daily smoking. This mental justification helps the smoker feel in control, as though they are somehow immune to the real risks. Yet the science is clear: occasional smoking, though less frequent, still exposes the lungs, heart, and bloodstream to the same toxic chemicals, leading to the same risks of cardiovascular disease, cancer, and respiratory issues.

Research underscores that there's no "safe" amount of exposure to tobacco smoke. Even one cigarette per day has been linked to a 50% increased risk of coronary heart disease compared to non-smokers, according to the British Medical Journal. Occasional smoking isn't a middle ground; it's a dangerous behaviour that straddles the same line as regular smoking, trading immediate health for short-lived social rewards. The brain's powerful reward system, coupled with the occasional smoker's cognitive dissonance, provides a perfect environment for addiction to flourish, silently transforming a "harmless" choice into a dangerous dependency.

The psychology behind occasional smoking reveals just how adept the brain is at self-deception. It wants pleasure, social connection, and a sense of control. But nicotine dependency undermines these desires, drawing the occasional smoker into a cycle they can't easily see or understand. The brain may rationalize occasional smoking as non-addictive, but each cigarette sends it deeper into the reward-seeking behaviours that drive addiction. This is how the myth of occasional smoking thrives, not because it's safe, but because our brains are wired to believe that it could be.

In the end, the myth of occasional smoking is just that, a myth, a false comfort in the face of an addictive substance that doesn't care how often it's used. Each cigarette reinforces the brain's craving for nicotine, laying down the neural pathways that can lead to dependency. And while the occasional smoker might feel immune, protected by infrequency, they're unknowingly caught in a mental and physical trap. For the brain, nicotine has no part-time contracts; every use is a reinforcement, every cigarette a step further down a path that could easily become permanent.

Behind the Smoke Veil

Let's pull back the curtain. Smoking addiction isn't just an accident. It's the result of careful, calculated design, a crafted trap engineered by one of the most manipulative industries in history. The cigarette you see isn't just a roll of tobacco. It's a meticulously designed instrument of dependency, one that's been perfected over decades to lock users in from the very first puff. With each inhalation, smokers aren't just consuming nicotine; they're fuelling an addiction created in a lab, one that has everything to do with profit and nothing to do with health or freedom.

It's no accident that nicotine is one of the most addictive substances on the planet. The tobacco industry knows this, and it's no secret that every cigarette is designed to deliver just the right amount to keep users hooked. The science here is clear: nicotine hijacks the brain's reward system, this hit is instant, surging within seconds of inhalation, creating a powerful association in the brain that links cigarettes with relief, pleasure, and satisfaction. But there's a catch, this satisfaction is short-lived. The brain soon craves another hit, another cigarette, and the cycle repeats. This is how dependency is engineered: through carefully controlled doses that create cravings almost as soon as they're satisfied. And as the smoker falls deeper into this dependency, each puff increases your speed down the *Cancer Highway*, and guess who hired the smartest engineers to make that road as appealing as it can be? None other than the tobacco industry.

But there's more to this engineered addiction than just nicotine. Over the years, tobacco companies have fine-tuned every element of the cigarette experience to hook users from the moment they open the box. Even the smell, the very first impression a smoker gets, is crafted to be appealing and enticing. The scent that escapes from a freshly opened pack isn't just random; it's deliberately formulated to create a powerful sensory association. In fact, research has shown that familiar smells can trigger cravings, prompting users to smoke even before the cigarette is lit. This tactic is subtle yet potent: by manipulating a sensory experience as basic as smell, tobacco companies create triggers that work on an almost unconscious level, priming the brain for addiction with every inhale.

And if you think these are unintentional consequences, think again. In the late 20th century, following strict advertising bans that cut off their access to traditional marketing, the tobacco industry didn't just shrink away. They adapted. They reinvented their strategy, shifting their focus to the cigarette itself. By modifying the product to intensify addiction, they ensured that smokers would come back regardless of ad campaigns. From adding chemicals that enhance nicotine's impact to adjusting the burn rate to maximize nicotine absorption, every aspect of the cigarette was refined to keep users dependent. This isn't marketing in the traditional sense; it's marketing through design, an approach that targets users at the most fundamental, biological level.

Even the cigarette's physical design is meant to manipulate. "Light" cigarettes, for example, were marketed as a safer alternative, a tactic that claimed to offer smokers a healthier choice. In reality, light cigarettes deliver nearly the same amount of tar and nicotine because smokers unknowingly take deeper drags to achieve the desired effect. The industry's own research showed that light cigarettes didn't reduce harm, but they continued to market them as a safe choice, preying on smokers' desires to quit or reduce harm. The truth is, there was never a safe cigarette, and these so-called alternatives only served to deepen addiction under the guise of "healthier" options.

And as the pressure mounted in the 1990s with lawsuits and increasing public scrutiny, the tobacco industry didn't change course, they just learned to get away with it better. To combat the growing body of evidence against them, tobacco companies invested heavily in funding biased studies that would paint a different picture. Through controlled studies designed to create conflicting data, they sowed seeds of doubt in the public mind, suggesting that smoking's dangers might not be as severe as critics claimed. By funding their own "research," they could control the narrative, presenting themselves as neutral entities and calling into question the findings of independent studies. This was not just a business decision, it was a deliberate campaign to obscure the truth, to cast a "smoke veil" over the dangers of smoking and maintain their stronghold on the market.

One notorious example of this tactic was the "Addiction Research Center" funded by tobacco giants to explore the supposed "safe use" of nicotine. This research was deeply flawed from the start, selectively choosing participants and methods to skew results in favour of the tobacco industry's goals. The data suggested that smoking could be safely managed, perpetuating the myth that "light" or "occasional" smoking posed minimal risk. But when exposed, the study revealed an ugly truth: tobacco companies were willing to manufacture science that protected their profits, even at the cost of public health.

Did you know that gasoline once contained lead, a toxic element that poisoned our air and our bodies? The effects were devastating: developmental disabilities in new-borns, cognitive damage in children, and serious health issues across communities. For years, the oil industry dismissed the dangers, propping up fake studies to convince the public that leaded gasoline was safe. But one scientist, Dr. Clair Patterson, stood up against them, risking his career and reputation to expose the truth. Patterson fought tirelessly, often alone, against powerful interests, and by the narrowest margin, he succeeded in getting lead removed from gasoline, saving countless lives. Today, leaded gasoline is a thing of the past, a victory that highlights how dangerous corporate deception can be. Smoking is no different, a toxic habit we blindly pass around, harming ourselves and others. One day, future generations will look back and wonder: how did we willingly accept this?

The reality is, there was no depth to which these companies wouldn't sink. With billions at stake, they didn't just target smokers; they targeted non-smokers, too. Throughout the 1980s and 1990s, tobacco companies poured resources into creating brands and campaigns that specifically appealed to younger audiences. Colourful packaging, trendy designs, and a "cool" aesthetic were carefully constructed to attract younger, more impressionable consumers. And once they had smokers on the hook, they exploited this dependency ruthlessly. When smoking rates dropped in the West due to rising awareness, they shifted their focus to developing nations, where regulations were looser and where they could exploit populations with little access to the information that had started saving lives elsewhere. By marketing aggressively in countries with weaker restrictions, they created new markets to keep the profits flowing.

Understanding these tactics is crucial. Behind every cigarette lies a calculated decision, a choice to prioritize profit over people. And for smokers, especially those who genuinely want to quit, knowing the extent of this manipulation can be a powerful motivator. This industry was built on lies, carefully constructed to create dependency while hiding behind a veneer of "choice" and "freedom." But for the millions who try to quit each year, that choice is compromised by an industry that stacked the deck from the start, embedding addiction into every aspect of the product.

So, what can we do with this information? First, awareness. Every smoker deserves to know the truth, that their struggle to quit isn't about weakness or lack of willpower. It's about facing a substance that was deliberately engineered to be as addictive as possible. The science of dependency was weaponized by the tobacco industry, creating a product so powerful that it could override a person's natural inclinations, their health, and even their will to quit. Knowing this is the first step to breaking free.

Secondly, we need to hold these companies accountable. For decades, they have manipulated data, skewed research, and exploited the most vulnerable populations to protect their profits. Public awareness, coupled with firm regulatory actions, is essential to dismantling the tactics that have kept this deadly industry alive for so long. Only when we confront these corporations head-on, exposing their lies and demanding transparency, can we hope to curb the reach of smoking and its devastating effects.

Finally, let's recognize the power of collective action. Each person who chooses not to start, who decides to quit, or who supports someone in their journey to quit, chips away at the foundations of an industry that has preyed on our vulnerabilities. By educating ourselves and sharing the truth, we can create a culture where smoking is no longer seen as a harmless choice, but as a dangerous dependency fuelled by corporate greed, and hopefully, not too long from now, to put an end to this industry once and for all.

The *Cancer Highway* is ominous and overpowering, the fog blinds us and prevents us to see that there IS a way to slow down and to stop your journey before the fateful end of this path.

Part 3: Ending the Journey – A Smoke-Free Future

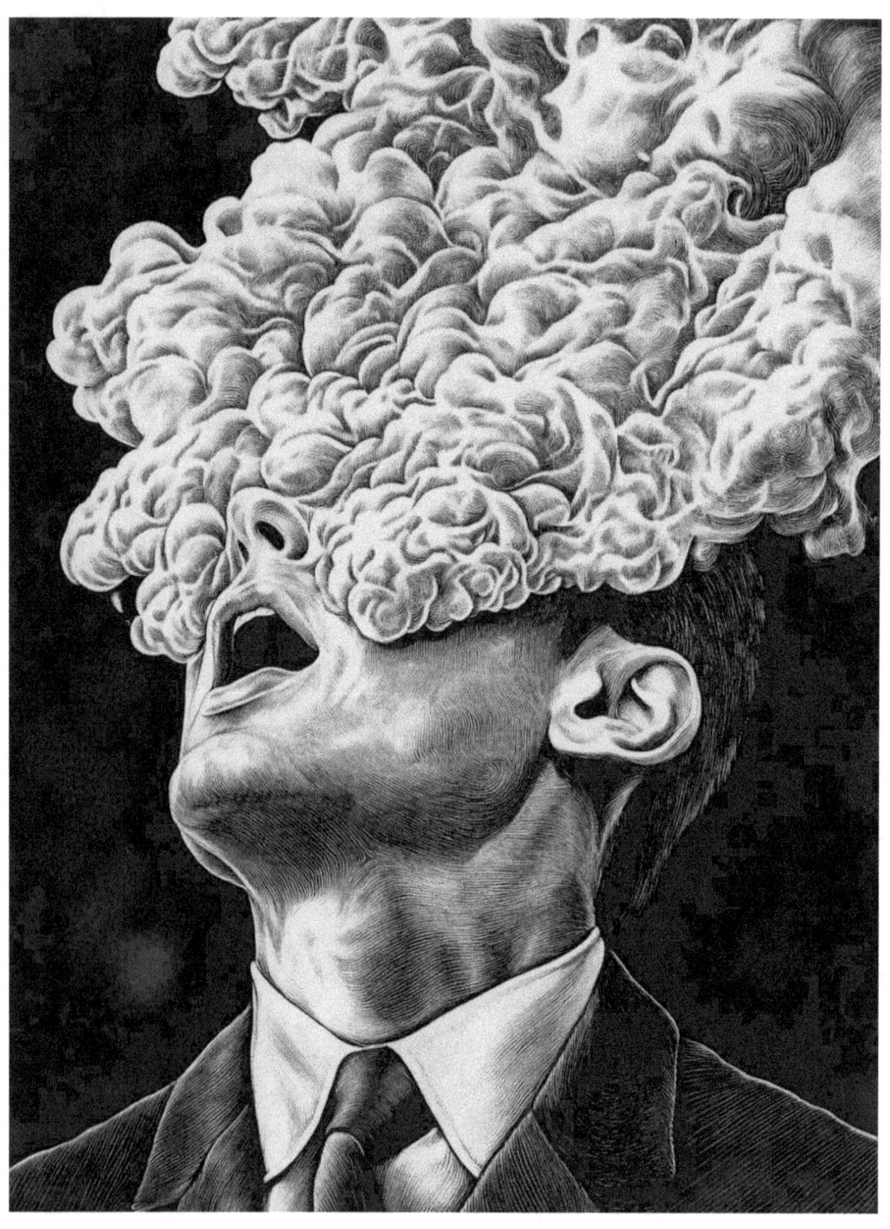

Chapter 6 | Expanding Smoke-Free Zones – Redrawing the Line

W here do you draw the line when it comes to self-preservation? It's a question that many of us rarely confront directly, but it's one worth considering. If you knew that your actions were putting you in danger, physically, mentally, or emotionally, would you stop? Or would you continue, aware of the consequences but hoping that the worst will never happen? How much self-harm is acceptable before it becomes a point of condemnation?

People tend to think of self-harm in extreme terms: dangerous physical behaviours, life-threatening situations, or destructive decisions that bring immediate consequences. But the reality is that many of the most harmful things we do to ourselves unfold slowly, often without us even realizing it. Slow-progressing harmful habits, such as smoking, poor diet, neglecting mental health, or engaging in toxic relationships, don't seem dangerous in the moment. There's no immediate fallout, no drastic change that forces us to stop and reconsider. So, we keep going, ignoring the subtle signs of harm, convincing ourselves that we'll deal with it later. But what happens when "later" becomes too late?

The human mind is particularly skilled at rationalizing these slow-moving threats. We tell ourselves that one more drink, one more cigarette, one more sleepless night won't really matter. After all, it hasn't caught up with us yet. It's easy to put off worrying about tomorrow when today feels manageable. Yet, as time goes on, these small acts of neglect accumulate, silently eroding our well-being. And too often, we only take things seriously when the consequences are irreversible, when the damage is done and our ability to undo it is lost.

Consider this: how much harm do we tolerate before we finally take action? And why do we so often wait until the damage is staring us in the face to make changes? Is it because the harm feels distant, abstract, or simply inconvenient to deal with? Maybe it's because we don't like to think about ourselves as being fragile or vulnerable. Admitting that we need to stop, or worse, change; feels like admitting weakness, so we push forward, ignoring the quiet alarms going off in the background.

But at what cost?

The real question is, **what is your limit?** At what point do you take the warning signs seriously and make a change before it's too late? The line between self-preservation and self-destruction is often thinner than we realize. By the time we recognize it, we may already be dangerously close to crossing it. So, where do you draw the line? How much harm will you accept before you take action, and what will it take to make you stop and protect yourself before it's too late?

Where We've Come So Far

The world today already looks very different from the time when smoking was not only accepted but glorified. There was a time when cigarettes were an accessory in every boardroom, every bar, and even hospitals. Smoking was embedded into everyday life, and the idea of restricting it seemed almost laughable. But, as we became more informed about the dangers of smoking, particularly second-hand smoke, public attitudes shifted, and so did the laws. What we've achieved since those smoke-filled days is nothing short of remarkable.

In the last few decades, the rise of indoor smoking bans has been one of the most significant public health victories across the globe. The ripple effects of these restrictions have reached nearly every corner of society, reshaping our norms and expectations of what it means to share public spaces. These bans didn't come overnight, they followed years of growing evidence about the devastating impact of all levels of smoking.

In the United States, a pivotal moment came in the 1990s when cities and states began enacting laws that banned smoking in public indoor spaces such as restaurants, bars, and workplaces. California was the first U.S. state to enact a comprehensive indoor smoking ban in 1995. It was revolutionary at the time, and yet, it set the stage for a wave of similar laws across the country. Today, 28 states have comprehensive smoke-free laws, and more than 80% of the U.S. population is protected by some form of smoke-free regulation.

Across the Atlantic, the United Kingdom followed a similar trajectory, though a few years behind. The landmark smoking ban in enclosed public spaces came into effect in 2007. Despite initial pushback, especially from pub and bar owners, the results have been striking. Air quality improved dramatically, and hospital admissions for heart attacks dropped within just a year of the ban's introduction. It wasn't just a public health success; it became a turning point in how society viewed smoking.

In both the U.S. and U.K., the bans were part of a broader societal shift, a move from viewing smoking as a personal choice to recognizing it as a public health threat. The damage smoking does isn't just to the smoker but to anyone who happens to be nearby. Second-hand smoke, which contains over 7,000 chemicals (including hundreds that are toxic and around 70 known carcinogens), became the focal point of the anti-smoking movement. Indoor bans were a way to protect the innocent, and in many ways, they succeeded. But while these laws changed the way we live indoors, the fight against smoking is far from over.

The indoor bans, as ground-breaking as they were, only addressed part of the problem. As smoking moved outside, the conversation shifted to what comes next. Now, the debate is heating up over whether outdoor smoking should be restricted as well. In the U.S. and the U.K., discussions are taking place about extending smoke-free zones to include parks, beaches, outdoor cafes, and even entire city centres.

The reasoning is simple: while outdoor spaces offer more ventilation than indoor ones, second-hand smoke remains a significant hazard. Outdoor smoking, especially in crowded areas like bus stops, playgrounds, and stadiums, continues to expose non-smokers to harmful chemicals. Studies have shown that in certain outdoor settings, such as patios or areas with restricted airflow, the level of exposure to second-hand smoke can be just as dangerous as indoors.

At the writing of this book, in the United States, cities like New York and San Francisco have been leading the charge, imposing bans on smoking in parks, on beaches, and at outdoor events. The city of Beverly Hills, California, went even further in 2019, implementing one of the country's most comprehensive bans on smoking in nearly all public spaces, both indoors and outdoors. This includes sidewalks, public buildings, and even multi-unit housing. It's a model that many other U.S. cities are watching closely as they consider expanding their own smoke-free policies.

In the United Kingdom, the debate has been similarly charged. London has been at the centre of calls to ban smoking in more outdoor areas, with growing support for making outdoor dining areas smoke-free. Wales has already implemented a ban on smoking in outdoor hospital grounds and school grounds, setting the stage for further restrictions.

These ongoing discussions are vital because they're not just about the individual rights of smokers. They're about the collective rights of the public, the right to breathe clean air, free from harmful toxins. The question of whether smoking in public should be allowed at all is becoming less of a fringe idea and more of a legitimate public health concern.

While the U.S. and U.K. are engaged in these debates, other countries have already forged ahead, setting examples of what might come next. One of the most striking examples is Australia, which has some of the toughest smoking laws in the world. Not only has the country banned smoking in most indoor public spaces, but it has also taken aggressive steps to restrict outdoor smoking. In Sydney, for example, smoking is banned in outdoor dining areas, at sports stadiums, and even within 10 meters of a playground. The result has been a dramatic reduction in smoking rates and a cultural shift away from the once-common sight of people smoking in public spaces.

New Zealand has taken things even further, with the government declaring smoking free status in 2025. This ambitious goal included phasing out the sale of cigarettes entirely for future generations. Their laws already ban smoking in most public outdoor spaces, and the country is pushing ahead with policies designed to eliminate smoking altogether.

In Japan, a country once notorious for high smoking rates, recent years have seen a significant clampdown on smoking in public spaces. With the 2020 Tokyo Olympics as a catalyst, the country imposed sweeping bans on smoking in restaurants, bars, and public spaces, even outdoors. The cultural shift in Japan is particularly noteworthy, given how entrenched smoking was in daily life. Now, smoking in public has become much less visible, and non-smokers are being given more protection from second-hand smoke.

These global examples demonstrate that stricter smoking laws are not only possible but effective. They provide a roadmap for countries like the U.S. and U.K., where outdoor smoking bans are still a topic of heated debate. But the direction is clear, countries that have taken stronger action are seeing the benefits, both in terms of public health and societal norms.

By the time of you reading this book, all that have been mentioned above could already be history, but much still has to happen for a whole world free of smoke.

So where have we come so far? The progress we've made is undeniable. Smoking, once an omnipresent part of daily life, is now something largely relegated to the margins. Indoor smoking bans have transformed our work-places, restaurants, and public spaces into cleaner, healthier environments. In many places, lighting up a cigarette in a public indoor space is not only illegal, it's unthinkable.

The reduction in smoking rates in countries like the U.S., the U.K., and Australia has been significant. In the U.S., smoking rates have plummeted from 42% in the 1960s to around 12.5% today. In the U.K., smoking prevalence has dropped to 14%, and the country is aiming for a smoke-free generation by 2030. These statistics are the result of sustained public health efforts, education, and legislation.

But this progress is just the beginning. Indoor smoking bans were the first major step in addressing the harms of tobacco, but they didn't solve the problem entirely. Smoking remains one of the leading causes of preventable death worldwide, and second-hand smoke continues to endanger the lives of non-smokers, especially in outdoor settings.

As the conversation shifts towards expanding smoke-free zones, it's clear that we're at a crossroads. The question is no longer whether smoking is harmful, we've known that for decades. The question now is: how much more can we do to protect people from its dangers? The answer lies in bold, decisive action that prioritizes public health over personal habit, drawing the line firmly between freedom and harm.

What Comes Next

The time has come to reconsider the concept of designated smoking areas entirely. Many hospitality settings, pubs, bars, and restaurants, still maintain these not-at-all-private zones reserved for smokers, even as the world grows increasingly smoke-free. But the truth is, these designated areas often fail to fully protect non-smokers from exposure. Smoke drifts, and the health consequences don't respect the boundaries of designated zones. Even if you're sitting on the "non-smoking" side of an outdoor patio, you will still be inhaling toxic fumes.

The argument for eliminating designated smoking areas is compelling. We know that exposure to second-hand smoke increases the risk of heart disease, lung cancer, and respiratory infections, even at low levels. The World Health Organization has made it clear that there is no safe level of exposure to tobacco smoke. So why do we allow spaces to exist where this exposure is practically guaranteed? Even if you, as a business owner, does not care if the customers are exposed to it, you are putting your staff at danger. Perhaps business should be more liable for exposing their staff in that manner, alike being liable for inappropriate handling of chemicals in the workplace, or contamination of any kind.

Australia and New Zealand are showing us by example the benefits of having stricter laws, and the results have been positive. Public support for such measures is growing, and businesses have adapted without significant loss of revenue. In fact, some studies suggest that smoke-free environments are more appealing to patrons, leading to increased foot traffic.

It's time to rethink what we accept as "normal" in public spaces. Smoking areas, whether indoors or outdoors, should no longer be a compromise. They are relics of a time when smoking was abundant, and their elimination is a logical step in the ongoing effort to prioritise public health.

Workplaces and educational institutions are another battleground in the fight against smoking. Smoke breaks have long been accepted as a necessary allowance for those who need a cigarette to get through the day, but they are more than just a moment of personal respite. They perpetuate the normalisation of smoking and create environments where non-smokers are often exposed to second-hand smoke, whether they want to be or not.

The argument against smoke breaks is not just about health; it's about fairness. Why should employees who smoke receive additional time away from their duties, while their non-smoking colleagues remain at their desks? In some cases, the cumulative time lost to smoke breaks can add up to hours each week, creating a disparity in productivity and work ethic.

In universities and colleges, where young adults are often making lifestyle choices that will follow them into adulthood, smoke breaks send the wrong message. Educational institutions should be environments that promote health and well-being, not places where tobacco and vaping use are quietly condoned through designated smoking areas or lenient policies. The removal of smoke breaks and smoking areas would signal a firm stance that smoking is not a behaviour to be accommodated or encouraged.

Many workplaces have already taken the initiative to implement smoke-free policies, and the trend is gaining momentum. As these policies become more widespread, the expectation will shift, and smoking at work will become as outdated as lighting up in an office meeting.

At home, one of the most urgent and complex issues in the future of smoking bans is the question of multi-family or multiple-occupancy housing. For non-smokers who live in apartment buildings or shared housing, second-hand smoke is not just an occasional nuisance; it can be a daily health hazard. Smoke seeps through walls, ventilation systems, and windows, meaning that even if you don't smoke, your neighbour's habit could still put you and your family at risk.

The science here is clear: second-hand smoke can travel in ways that are impossible to fully prevent without banning smoking in multi-unit housing altogether. This is particularly concerning for families with children, the elderly, and individuals with pre-existing health conditions. For them, living next to a smoker is not just unpleasant, it's dangerous.

Cities like Beverly Hills have already implemented stringent policies that ban smoking in all multi-unit housing, and it's time for other cities and countries to follow suit. Critics may argue that such bans infringe on personal freedom within one's home, but the right to smoke should not supersede the right of others to live in a smoke-free environment.

None of these changes will happen without strong, decisive action from governments. Public health campaigns, funded and supported by government initiatives, have been instrumental in reducing smoking rates worldwide. But there is more to be done, especially when it comes to confronting the tobacco industry itself.

Governments must take a firmer stand against tobacco companies, which continue to market their deadly products, often targeting vulnerable populations. This includes not only implementing stricter regulations on advertising and sales but also increasing funding for quitting smoking programs. These programs have proven to be effective, but they need to be accessible, affordable, and widely promoted.

The future of smoking bans will not be defined by individual action alone; it will require a concerted effort from governments, communities, and health advocates to continue pushing for a world where smoking is no longer the norm. In many ways, the groundwork has already been laid. We have seen how effective smoke-free policies can be in reducing smoking rates and improving public health. The next step is to extend those protections to everyone, in every space, indoors and out, public and private.

In the end, the goal is clear: a future where the harmful effects of smoking are no longer tolerated, where clean air is a right, not a privilege, and where the freedom to live a healthy life outweighs the freedom to smoke. The time for half-measures is over. The future demands bold action, and it's up to all of us to make it happen.

Chapter 7 | Changing Minds – Pulling up the hand break

G aslighting is a psychological tactic that has gained notoriety in recent years, although its origins stretch back far beyond the term itself. At its core, gaslighting is a method of manipulation in which the perpetrator seeks to make the target doubt their perceptions, memories, or even sanity. It is a slow, insidious process, one that erodes the victim's sense of reality and renders them more vulnerable to the manipulator's influence. This concept goes beyond personal relationships, it extends into broader societal dynamics, where companies and people in power use it to manipulate public opinion, skew reality, and entrench their authority.

The term "gaslighting" comes from the 1938 play *Gas Light*, and later the 1944 film adaptation, where a husband systematically manipulates his wife into believing she is losing her mind by altering her environment in subtle ways, such as dimming the gas lights, then denying the changes. Over time, his wife begins to question her own perceptions and judgments, growing increasingly dependent on her husband's narrative of events.

At its essence, gaslighting relies on exploiting the inherent vulnerabilities of the human mind. It works by gradually undermining a person's confidence in their own thoughts, leading them to accept an alternate, false version of reality. The brilliance, and the danger, of gaslighting lies in its subtlety. The manipulator doesn't confront the victim with overt lies, but rather, they present a series of half-truths, distortions, and contradictions that sow confusion and self-doubt. Once doubt sets in, the gaslighter becomes a point of reference, the arbiter of what is "real."

The human mind is remarkably adept at absorbing information, yet it is also deeply flawed in its ability to process that information rationally, especially when under stress or uncertainty. Psychologists have long noted that our memories are malleable, our perceptions biased, and our reasoning subject to emotional influences. In fact, our minds are wired to prioritize coherence and cognitive ease over factual accuracy. This creates fertile ground for manipulation.

Cognitive biases, such as confirmation bias, make it easier for us to accept information that aligns with our existing beliefs, while discrediting information that contradicts them. This tendency makes gaslighting especially effective because the victim may cling to any glimmer of hope that aligns with their desire for reassurance, even if it means accepting falsehoods. Furthermore, people tend to prefer social harmony and may conform to the opinions of others to avoid conflict or ostracization. Gaslighters exploit this human need for consensus by presenting their false narratives as the dominant, socially accepted view.

Studies in social psychology demonstrate how easily people can be manipulated through subtle cues and suggestions. The famous *Asch conformity experiments* conducted by psychologist Solomon Asch in 1950s, for example, showed that individuals would agree with a clearly incorrect answer just because others in the group had done so. Similarly, the *Stanford prison experiment* by Philip Zimbardo in 1971, revealed how quickly people could adopt abusive behaviours or subservient roles based on perceived authority. These experiments reflect the disturbing ease with which perception and behaviour can be influenced by external forces, whether those forces are individuals, groups, or institutions.

Gaslighting is not confined to personal interactions; it has been adopted by corporations, media outlets, and governments as a tool for controlling narratives and shaping public perception. In many cases, it is done with a level of sophistication that is almost invisible to the average person, embedded in the flow of information we consume daily.

Corporate entities, for instance, have long used gaslighting techniques to influence consumer behaviour, like a spell of sorts. Consider the tobacco industry's decades-long effort to deny the link between smoking and lung cancer. Despite overwhelming scientific evidence, tobacco companies created doubt through misleading studies, paid experts, and targeted PR campaigns. By distorting the truth and casting doubt on credible research, they were able to manipulate public opinion and delay regulatory action. This form of corporate gaslighting exploits the human tendency to believe authority figures and rely on "expert" opinions, even when those opinions are manipulated.

Breaking the Spell

For generations, the habit bound smokers in a spell. It was more than just a habit, it was an image, a persona, a lifestyle. Think back to the black-and-white movies where screen legends leaned back, blowing plumes of smoke into the air with a casual elegance, or the Marlboro Man, that tough, rugged cowboy who made cigarettes seem like a symbol of freedom and independence. The tobacco industry spent billions of dollars weaving smoking into the fabric of everyday life, making it appear like a rite of passage or a mark of adulthood. But behind this illusion, there was always a darker reality. Beneath the glamour was a slow march towards disease, dependency, and death. If you don't know how Marlboro Man spent his last years on earth, I suggest you look at it.

Breaking the spell wasn't easy. For decades, the tobacco industry fought tooth and nail to protect the illusion that smoking was harmless, even desirable. But then came the counterattack, the rise of anti-smoking campaigns that pulled back the curtain and showed the world what smoking really does. At the heart of this movement were campaigns like "Truth," a powerful force that began reshaping how we view smoking.

The *Truth* campaign was, in many ways, a game-changer. It didn't rely on the typical anti-smoking messages that people had grown numb to. It wasn't just another lecture on how smoking causes lung cancer or heart disease, although those facts remain central. Instead, *Truth* tapped into something deeper: it attacked the very foundation of the tobacco industry's marketing, its manipulation, its deceit, and its exploitation of young people. By the time *Truth* launched in the early 2000s, tobacco companies had spent decades building brands that seduced the public with the promise of something better: more style, more confidence, more social acceptance. But *Truth* flipped that narrative on its head.

Through a series of clever and provocative ads, *Truth* targeted young people with messages that exposed the tobacco industry's lies. Rather than simply telling teens that smoking was bad, *Truth* made it about rebellion. It painted smoking as a corporate trap, a way for the industry to line its pockets while knowingly pushing a product that killed. It was no longer about smoking being uncool, it was about standing up to an industry that didn't care if you lived or died as long as you kept buying their cigarettes.

One of *Truth*'s most iconic ads featured young activists placing body bags outside a major tobacco company's headquarters, a stark reminder of the millions of lives lost to cigarettes each year. It wasn't just a fear tactic, it was a wake-up call. The campaign didn't blame smokers for their addiction; instead, it exposed the powerful machine that made people addicted in the first place. This approach resonated deeply, particularly with younger audiences who had grown up questioning authority and corporate motives. Smoking, in the eyes of many, became not a personal choice but a social injustice.

And the numbers proved it worked. Teen smoking rates in the United States dropped dramatically, and much of that decline was credited to *Truth*'s innovative strategies. Between 2000 and 2002 alone, youth smoking rates fell by 23%, a staggering victory in the fight against tobacco.

But while *Truth* was reshaping public opinion through smart, youth-oriented messaging, another tool in the battle against smoking was gaining ground: graphic warnings on cigarette packs. If *Truth* used strategy and wit to dismantle the appeal of smoking, graphic warnings went straight for the gut, forcing smokers to confront the terrifying physical consequences of their habit every time they reached for a cigarette.

Introduced in countries around the world, these warnings featured grue-some, unfiltered images, blackened lungs, cancerous mouths, decaying teeth, and dead bodies. They were stark, shocking, and impossible to ignore. Unlike the text warnings of the past, which many smokers grew accustomed to tuning out, these new warnings were visceral and inescapable. In Canada, the introduction of graphic warnings led to a significant increase in quit attempts, with 31% of smokers admitting that the images made them consider giving up cigarettes. In Australia, where graphic warnings were paired with plain packaging that stripped cigarette boxes of all branding, smoking rates plummeted. Without the glossy marketing to hide behind, cigarettes became what they truly are: symbols of death and disease.

While these graphic warnings were controversial, with some critics arguing they relied too heavily on fear, the evidence showed they were effective. Studies across multiple countries confirmed that the images made smokers more likely to quit and less likely to start in the first place. They also sent a strong message to potential smokers, particularly younger people: smoking isn't glamorous or cool, it's a fast track to a hospital bed or a coffin.

What made these warnings so powerful was that they shattered the carefully crafted illusion that the tobacco industry had spent decades building. Cigarette packs, once designed to be sleek and appealing, now carried the blunt truth of what their product does. It was a psychological shift that forced even the most hardened smokers to confront the reality of their addiction. You couldn't escape it. Every time you bought a pack, there it was: a reminder that smoking leads to cancer, disfigurement, and death. And while some smokers grew desensitised to the images over time, for many, it was the nudge they needed to finally quit.

But the battle didn't end with shock tactics and anti-industry messaging. The key to truly breaking the spell of smoking was changing the narrative altogether. Smoking could no longer be seen as a personal choice that only affected the individual. It had to be seen for what it really is: a public health crisis, a societal burden, and an epidemic driven by corporate greed.

By reframing smoking as a moral and social issue, public health campaigns were able to garner wider support for stricter regulations, higher taxes on tobacco products, and smoking bans in public spaces. Governments around the world began to take more aggressive steps to curb smoking rates, realising that the cost of tobacco addiction, both in lives lost and healthcare expenses, was too high to ignore.

And yet, breaking the spell isn't just about stopping smoking, it's about preventing it from ever starting again. As new generations grow up in a world where smoking is increasingly stigmatised and regulated, it's easy to forget just how powerful the tobacco industry's hold once was. The fight isn't over, but these campaigns have made significant strides. They've helped dismantle the glamorous facade that once surrounded smoking, replacing it with a more accurate, and far less appealing, image.

The spell that smoking cast for so long is cracking. The *Truth* campaign, graphic warnings, and the ongoing efforts to raise awareness have all played a role in pulling back the curtain. People now know the reality: smoking kills, and it's not something to be admired or emulated. It's something to be avoided at all costs. And while tobacco companies will continue to fight for their survival, the tide has shifted. The question is no longer whether smoking is harmful, that's been settled. The question now is how fast we can rid society of this deadly habit once and for all.

But as we look towards the future, the battle is shifting into new territories, especially the digital world, where the influence of social media is shaping new generations' opinions on what's "cool." The spell may be breaking, but there are new challenges ahead, and the fight to change minds is far from over.

The Role of The Social Media

In the fight against smoking, the battlefield has changed. Tobacco companies don't have a direct, visible, distinct hold on consumer as they used to have, everything is more nuanced nowadays. We are no longer just fighting cigarette companies through TV ads and health campaigns; now we're fighting on a new front: the social media. Social platforms like Instagram, TikTok, YouTube, and former Twitter have become the new arenas where culture is shaped, where trends are born, and where the youth spend hours of their day. If we want to break the hold that smoking and vaping have on people, especially younger generations, we have to meet them where they are. And today, they are online.

In a world where influencers, celebrities, and content creators shape so much of what we consider "cool" or desirable, social media holds immense power. It's no longer enough to just rely on public health campaigns or warning labels. If smoking and vaping are still seen as rebellious, fashionable, or even just normalised in the digital spaces that young people frequent, then the battle isn't truly won. We need to shift the narrative online, and that starts with the people who hold the most influence: the creators.

Imagine a 16-year-old scrolling through their TikTok feed. They come across their favourite influencer, someone with millions of followers, who seems to have it all: the looks, the lifestyle, the attention. And there, casually, is that influencer holding a vape or lighting up a cigarette in a video. The message is subtle, but it's powerful. Whether that creator is promoting smoking directly or not, they're still showing it to millions of impressionable followers. It's a quiet endorsement, and for some young viewers, it sends the message that smoking or vaping is just a part of the cool, carefree lifestyle they see on social media.

Ok, that was a little bit of an unlike scenario, TikTok currently have a stronger hold on promotion or glorification of smoking and vaping among minors, but not necessarily among adults, which, let's be honest, will be followed by minors. The enforcement of these rules is inconsistent at best.

This is where change has to happen. Influencers and celebrities have a responsibility, whether they realise it or not. With millions of eyes on them, their choices have ripple effects. If smoking or vaping is seen in their content, it normalises these habits. But if those same influencers actively promote smoke-free lifestyles, that message can spread just as quickly.

We've already seen how influencers can shape public opinion in areas like fitness, diet, and mental health. In recent years, platforms have been flooded with wellness content, meditation routines, yoga challenges, recipes for healthy eating. This trend has gained massive traction because influencers make it aspirational. They show their followers that taking care of your body and mind isn't just about health; it's about looking and feeling your best. Now, imagine if that same energy was directed towards promoting a smoke-free life. If influencers and celebrities who have huge followings start talking about why they don't smoke or vape, why they choose wellness over addiction, that could shift the conversation in a big way.

A few influencers and celebrities have already started speaking out about the dangers of smoking and vaping, but it's not nearly enough. There needs to be a larger movement, one that treats smoking and vaping like the outdated, unhealthy habits they are. Just as we've seen trends like clean eating and fitness challenges take over Instagram, there's potential for a similar push towards smoke-free living. But it has to start with the influencers who have the biggest platforms. They are the gatekeepers to the next generation's attitudes, and their voices carry weight.

But it's not just about promoting healthy living, it's about being honest about the harms of smoking when it does appear, if even. If an influencer or someone in the background is smoking or vaping in their content, there should be no room for ambiguity. There needs to be a push for automatic disclaimers when addictive habits are depicted in videos or posts. Just like we now see labels on paid promotions or sponsored content, there should be a disclaimer that reminds viewers of the risks associated with smoking or vaping. This doesn't have to be invasive, but it should be clear enough to remind people that these habits are dangerous.

The goal here isn't to shame individuals for smoking or vaping, but to ensure that when these habits are shown, the risks are never forgotten. Too often, social media glosses over the reality of addiction. A quick video showing someone puffing on a vape doesn't show the long-term health effects. It doesn't show the dependency or the damage to lungs. Disclaimers would help ensure that viewers don't see smoking or vaping as just another harmless activity.

One of the most effective ways to change behaviour on social media is by targeting creators' financial incentives. Right now, a video featuring smoking or vaping could be monetised just like any other content. Creators can get paid for ads running alongside videos that normalise or glamorise these habits.

That needs to change. There should be stricter monetisation rules on social media platforms that prohibit content creators from profiting off the depiction of smoking or vaping.

This already happens in other areas. Content that features violence or explicit material often gets age-restricted or demonetised. The same should apply to smoking and vaping. If creators knew they couldn't earn money from videos that show or promote these habits, it would likely reduce the amount of such content on their channels. If platforms like YouTube, TikTok, and Instagram enforced these rules, it would send a strong message: smoking and vaping aren't trends we want to encourage, and there's no financial reward for doing so.

If there's one thing that social media excels at, it's turning trends into status symbols. Over the past few years, we've seen wellness become the ultimate aspirational lifestyle. Influencers post about their plant-based diets, their rigorous workout routines, and their dedication to self-care. Clean living has become the gold standard of success. This is a powerful shift, and it's one we can build on in the fight against smoking.

What if, instead of seeing vaping devices in influencers' hands, we saw them embracing everyday healthy habits, like drinking water, taking a walk in the park, or preparing a simple home-cooked meal? What if, instead of romanticising late-night parties filled with smoke, we saw people enjoying relaxed, smoke-free get-togethers or just unwinding at home? Healthy living doesn't have to mean intense workouts or extreme diets, it's about making small, realistic choices that promote well-being. Social media could help reshape the idea of success, not as an unattainable ideal, but as a balanced lifestyle that values feeling good, both mentally and physically, in the everyday moments of life.

The beauty of this movement is that it doesn't have to be forced. Wellness is already popular. People are looking for ways to improve their health, feel better, and live longer. Influencers are capitalising on this trend, and it's only a matter of time before we see the same approach applied to smoking and vaping. By making clean living aspirational, we can start to chip away at the idea that smoking or vaping is edgy or glamorous. Instead, we can replace it with a new image, one where true success is measured by how well you take care of your body, not by the clouds of smoke you leave behind.

Ultimately, the role of social media in the fight against smoking can't be underestimated. It's where culture gets shaped, where trends are born, and where millions of people, especially young people, spend their time. If we want to truly break the cycle of smoking and vaping addiction, we need to harness the power of these platforms.

By pushing influencers and celebrities to promote smoke-free lifestyles, by demanding transparency and accountability in the content that gets posted, by introducing stricter monetisation rules, perhaps better rewards for healthier influences, and by making wellness and clean living the new status symbol, we can turn the tide. We've already seen what social media can do for fitness, nutrition, and mental health. It's time to use that same power to put an end to the social acceptability of smoking and vaping.

The old spell that smoking once cast has been broken in many ways, but in the digital age, we need new tools and strategies to fight back. The battle has moved online, and if we don't rise to the challenge, the next generation could continue to fall victim to the same mistakes of the past. Social media offers us an opportunity to change that narrative, for good. The question is: are people willing?

Chapter 8 | Holding the Tobacco Industry Accountable

Have you heard of the Tuskegee Syphilis Experiment? It's one of the most notorious examples of unethical medical research in American history. Conducted between 1932 and 1972, the Tuskegee Study of Untreated Syphilis in the Negro Male was a secretive clinical study carried out by the U.S. Public Health Service (PHS) and the Tuskegee Institute. The experiment involved 600 African American men from Alabama, 399 of whom had syphilis, while the remaining 201 served as a control group. The men were told they were being treated for "bad blood," a vague term covering a variety of ailments, but in reality, they were not being treated for syphilis at all.

The purpose of the study was to observe the natural progression of untreated syphilis, even though penicillin had become the standard and effective treatment for the disease by 1947. Despite this, the men in the Tuskegee experiment were deliberately denied access to this life-saving treatment, and many suffered severe health consequences, including blindness, mental illness, heart disease, and even death. Their families, too, suffered, with many wives contracting syphilis and children being born with congenital syphilis.

The study continued for 40 years before it was finally exposed to the public in 1972, thanks to a whistle-blower who leaked the information to the press. When the story broke, it caused national outrage. People were horrified to learn that such a cruel and deceptive study had been allowed to continue for so long, especially considering that it targeted a marginalized group already facing systemic racism and inequality in health care.

However, despite the public outrage, none of the individual researchers who were involved in the study faced legal consequences. The U.S. government eventually offered financial settlements to the victims and their families, but no one was ever prosecuted or held accountable for the gross violations of human rights that occurred during the study.

How do you feel about that? Shouldn't there be consequences when professionals in positions of trust abuse their power and inflict harm on vulnerable populations? The Tuskegee experiment is often held up as a shocking reminder of the lengths to which institutions can go in exploiting human lives for some sort of gain, particularly when those lives belong to marginalized communities.

Some argue that the lack of legal consequences for those involved in Tuskegee is a stain on America's medical and legal systems. They question how such an atrocity could go unpunished, even after it was exposed. Others point to the fact that systemic racism made it easier for these abuses to take place, and harder for justice to be served afterward. The damage was done, lives were destroyed, yet no one was held responsible.

Sadly, history often repeats itself. Today, as the world grapples with new threats to global health, many people wonder if those in positions of power and responsibility will once again escape accountability. Are we seeing another chapter of negligence or exploitation that no one will be held responsible for? Health crises, misinformation, and unethical practices still exist, and many wonder whether those behind these failures will ever face justice.

Exposing the Industry's Tactics

The tobacco industry has played us all for fools for decades. This is no conspiracy theory. It's a well-documented fact that the corporations behind cigarettes and vapes have systematically manipulated their products, their marketing, and the truth, all in the name of profit. The tactics they use are nothing short of sinister, and the damage they've caused is staggering.

First, let's talk about how they market addiction. It sounds brutal, but that's exactly what they do. There's no way around it: promoted through subtle but powerful psychological tactics. From the very beginning, the goal wasn't just to sell a product; it was to hook people on it for life. Nicotine is, as I have previously mentioned, one of the most addictive substances on the planet, comparable to heroin and cocaine. The industry has known this for over half a century and still chose to engineer cigarettes that would make quitting near impossible.

They've done it through manipulation, starting with what's inside the product itself. You know now that cigarettes are chemically designed to deliver nicotine to the brain faster and more efficiently, ensuring a quicker and deeper addiction. Once someone starts smoking, the cravings take over and keep them coming back, no matter the consequences to their health. It's no accident that many smokers light up their first cigarette as teenagers; this is a calculated move. Tobacco companies have historically targeted young people, knowing that the younger someone starts, the harder it will be for them to quit. Get them addicted young, and they'll likely be customers for life, or until the addiction kills them.

Then, there's the manipulation of public perception. For decades, tobacco companies poured money into marketing campaigns designed to downplay the dangers of smoking. They sponsored glamorous Hollywood movies, showed attractive, successful people smoking in advertisements, and linked cigarettes to freedom, rebellion, or even fitness, anything but the deadly truth. Early on, cigarette ads featured doctors endorsing brands, giving the impression that smoking was harmless, even healthy. As ridiculous as that seems now, it worked. It's one of the most significant examples of corporate deception in modern history. I know I'm talking about something that happened in the past and is no longer acceptable, but is it even possible to calculate the long-term damage of those campaigns? Could they still be influencing people to this date?

Even when the scientific community began to reach an undeniable consensus about the health risks of smoking, Big Tobacco wasn't willing to back down. In fact, they doubled down. They employed so-called "experts" and lobbyists to create doubt, to keep the public confused about the dangers of their products. They sowed uncertainty, much like the fossil fuel industry has done with climate change, making it seem like the risks of smoking were still up for debate. The infamous "Frank Statement" of the 1950s, where tobacco companies openly denied the health risks of their products, was a blatant lie that delayed meaningful action for years.

While the public was slowly waking up to the dangers of smoking, the tobacco industry continued its assault through aggressive lobbying. They fought tooth and nail against regulations that would reduce smoking rates or restrict their marketing. They targeted politicians and lawmakers with millions in campaign contributions, pushing back against every attempt to introduce legislation that might make it harder to sell cigarettes. For decades, they were largely successful, blocking efforts to regulate tobacco as a harmful substance and avoiding the restrictions placed on other dangerous products.

Even today, their tactics haven't disappeared. They've just evolved. Enter the era of e-cigarettes and vapes, a product that was originally touted as a safer alternative to traditional smoking, even a tool to help people quit. But let's be honest, vaping has turned into a whole new way for the industry to hook the next generation. Instead of cigarettes, today's teens are reaching for vapes, often under the impression that it's harmless. Spoiler alert: it's not.

Vape companies, which are often owned by the same big tobacco corporations, have employed the same marketing tactics that worked so well for cigarettes. Flashy ads, influencer campaigns, and a whole range of sweet, fruity flavours designed to appeal to young people. They've even gone as far as to suggest that vaping is a form of harm reduction, which is a dangerously misleading narrative. Yes, vaping might be less harmful than smoking traditional cigarettes, but that doesn't mean it's safe. And what's most alarming is the growing evidence that vaping is just as effective as cigarettes in creating a new generation of nicotine addicts, perhaps more because it is far more accessible to children and teenagers than cigarettes ever were.

Big Tobacco hasn't just been sitting back and letting regulation happen either. No, they've been actively fighting against it at every step, particularly in low- and middle-income countries where tobacco use is still rising. They push back on efforts to implement higher taxes, restrict advertising, or introduce plain packaging. They target vulnerable governments with legal threats and economic pressure, ensuring that they can continue to profit off addiction, regardless of the cost in human lives. In some cases, they've even taken governments to court to block anti-smoking laws, prioritising corporate profits over public health.

It is hard to believe, but there are still countries where the usage of tobacco is growing due to lack of laws and regulations to prevent it. Countries like Congo, Egypt, Indonesia, Jordan, Oman and Moldova. Indonesia in particular continues to have one of the world's highest smoking rates, over 70% of adult males are smokers. This is solely due to the aggressive marketing still allowed in the country.

The reality is this: the tobacco industry has built a vast empire on the backs of addiction and disease. It's an industry that thrives on keeping people hooked, regardless of the consequences. And as much as they try to hide behind claims of personal responsibility, the truth is that they've spent billions engineering a product that is designed to be impossible to quit. That's not personal choice. That's manipulation on a massive scale.

So, what do we do about it? We expose these tactics for what they are: calculated moves to keep people addicted, to keep profits flowing, and to keep the truth buried. We shine a light on the fact that the tobacco industry has repeatedly lied, manipulated, and resisted change, all to protect their bottom line. We hold them accountable for the damage they've done, not just to the millions of people who have died because of their products, but to the families left behind, the health systems burdened by the cost of treating smoking-related diseases, and the billions in lost productivity.

It's time to stop treating tobacco companies like any other business. This isn't an industry that makes harmless products for consumers to choose from. This is an industry built on addiction, disease, and death, and it needs to be held to account for the lives it has destroyed. Holding the tobacco industry accountable starts with recognising the truth: they are selling death, and they've been lying about it for decades. Now, it's time to turn the tide, expose their tactics, and demand justice for the generations they have harmed.

Increased Taxes and Penalties

If we're serious about reducing smoking rates and holding the tobacco industry accountable, we have to hit them where it hurts: their wallets. Increased taxes and penalties are among the most effective tools we have to make smoking financially unsustainable, not just for individual smokers, but for the industry as a whole.

Let's start with the simplest and most proven strategy: raising taxes. There's no question about it, higher tobacco taxes save lives. Study after study shows that when the price of cigarettes goes up, smoking rates go down, especially among young people and low-income smokers. Why? Because tobacco is highly price-sensitive. Make it too expensive, and fewer people will start smoking, while others will be motivated to quit. It's one of the few policies where the benefits are both immediate and long-term.

But here's the thing: we're not talking about just a small bump in price. To make a real difference, taxes need to be significantly higher. Many countries have already seen success with steep tobacco taxes, but there's still room for more aggressive action, especially in places where tobacco products remain cheap and accessible. The tobacco industry will, of course, argue that this penalizes consumers, but the truth is, it's their addictive products that are trapping people in this cycle in the first place. High taxes are a way of forcing both smokers and the industry to pay for the immense damage smoking causes, damage that is usually footed by the public in terms of healthcare costs and lost productivity.

And we're not just talking about cigarettes. Vapes and e-cigarettes need to be taxed heavily too. While some argue that vaping is a less harmful alternative, the reality is that these products are still addictive and dangerous, particularly for younger generations. By raising the price of all nicotine products, we send a clear message: addiction isn't cheap, and the true cost of smoking and vaping needs to be reflected in their price tags.

Taxes are just one part of the solution. The tobacco industry also needs to be held legally accountable for the harm it's caused. Lawsuits are a powerful way to do this. We've seen landmark cases in the past where tobacco companies were ordered to pay massive settlements for lying about the dangers of smoking, concealing evidence, and marketing to minors. But the fight isn't over. There are still billions of dollars to be claimed in damages, especially as more evidence comes to light about the industry's deceptive practices.

Governments should continue to pursue these lawsuits aggressively. Every dollar that tobacco companies are forced to pay in damages is a dollar that can be used to fund anti-smoking campaigns, healthcare for smoking-related illnesses, and programs to help people quit. It also serves as a powerful deterrent—if the industry knows it will be hit with massive penalties every time it steps out of line, it will think twice before engaging in deceptive practices or trying to undermine public health regulations.

The tobacco industry has fought back against these lawsuits with all its might, employing teams of lawyers and lobbyists to delay justice. But persistence is key. The public has a right to seek reparations for the decades of harm caused by cigarettes and vapes. These lawsuits are not just about money; they're about justice for the millions of people who have suffered because of the industry's greed and lies.

Another important, yet often overlooked, way to tackle the tobacco epidemic is through travel restrictions. Cigarettes and vapes are too easy to smuggle across borders, especially through airports and checkpoints. To disrupt this flow, we need to implement stricter bans on transporting tobacco products through these channels.

Imagine a world where you can't casually bring cigarettes or vapes with you when traveling internationally or even domestically. If we ban the carrying of cigarettes and vapes through airports and border checks, we create another layer of difficulty for smokers and, more importantly, for those who attempt to distribute tobacco products illegally. This not only reduces access but also helps to clamp down on the illegal tobacco trade, which is another major source of revenue for the industry.

Additionally, implementing these travel restrictions sends a strong message: tobacco is no longer something we tolerate or treat as a normal consumer good. It's a toxic product that costs lives, and we should treat it with the same level of caution and control as other dangerous substances.

These travel bans would also have a powerful symbolic effect. Imagine walking through an airport and seeing it as a tobacco-free zone, not just smoke-free, but a place where cigarettes and vapes aren't allowed to pass through customs or boarding gates. It reinforces the idea that smoking is not just a personal choice but a public health crisis that demands bold action.

Beyond the immediate benefits of reducing smoking rates and protecting public health, these policies would have a long-term, crippling effect on the tobacco industry. Higher taxes, expensive lawsuits, and tighter restrictions would eat into the industry's profit margins, forcing them to either change their business model or pay for the harm they've caused.

This is important because as long as the tobacco industry is profitable, it will continue to find ways to sell its products and hook new customers. We've seen it happen before, every time smoking rates drop in one country, Big Tobacco shifts its focus to new markets, particularly in developing nations where regulations are weaker and smoking is still on the rise. By increasing the financial penalties for tobacco companies across the board, we can start to put a real dent in their bottom line, making it less attractive for them to continue operating as usual.

Let's put this in perspective. Every year, globally, about 97,000 people die from stabbings. Sugary drinks? They contribute to 180,000 deaths. Gun incidents claim 250,000 lives. HIV/AIDS takes around 650,000 people annually. Diabetes is responsible for 1.5 million deaths. And road-related accidents, cars, planes, pedestrians, cyclists, account for 1.9 million deaths worldwide. These are staggering numbers, but here's the kicker: cigarettes kill over 8 million people every single year. Let that sink in.

Despite this, no one bats an eyelid. We're all painfully aware of the other causes. We point fingers at the U.S. for its gun violence epidemic. In the UK, people are deeply concerned about rising stabbing deaths. But when it comes to smoking, a habit that poisons not just the smoker but everyone around them, children included, we've been conditioned to turn a blind eye. The manipulation runs deep. We're hyper-aware of other dangers, yet somehow, we've normalized a product that kills more people than any of them combined. That's the real tragedy.

In the end, this part of the battle comes down to one clear strategy: make smoking and vaping too expensive and legally risky to continue. Increased taxes will reduce consumption by making tobacco products unaffordable for many, while lawsuits and penalties will ensure that the industry pays for the damage it has caused. And by banning the transport of cigarettes and vapes through airports and border checks, we can disrupt the supply chain and send a strong message that the days of Big Tobacco profiting off addiction are numbered.

Currently, the price of cigarettes is nowhere near high enough to reflect the true cost of smoking. In the UK, a pack of cigarettes averages around £10, and in the U.S., it's roughly $7. That's a joke. Each cigarette in the UK costs about £0.50, pocket change for a product that's designed to kill you and those around you slowly. Those numbers should be much, much higher. There's no valid argument against pricing cigarettes out of existence. None. If a pack of cigarettes were £25 or £30, we'd be living in a healthier, better world. And if you think that's too expensive, think again.

In the UK, a night out at a restaurant can easily cost more than £30 per person. A single cinema ticket costs almost double what you currently pay for a pack of cigarettes. So, ask yourself, how does the cost of a pack of cigarettes compare to other everyday expenses where you live? Is smoking really cheaper than going out to dinner or catching a movie? It shouldn't be. Smoking is far deadlier, and it's time the price tag reflected that harsh reality.

The tobacco industry has gotten away with too much for too long. It's time for them to face real consequences, both financially and legally. Raising taxes and pushing for tougher penalties are the first steps toward a future where smoking is not just a dangerous habit but an unsustainable one.

Chapter 9 | Supporting Smokers to Quit – Compassionate but Firm Solutions

L et's talk about quitting. Not the vague "yeah, I should probably stop someday" quitting, but real, hard quitting, the type that's backed by proper support and solid, accessible programs. Quitting smoking isn't about sheer willpower. Sure, determination plays a role, but when you're facing a habit as insidious and gripping as smoking, it's like trying to climb a mountain without the right gear. Smokers deserve the best equipment to help them get out of this battle, and that means quit programs need to be accessible to all, no exceptions.

Quit Programs for All

In an ideal world, everyone who wanted to quit smoking would have a well-stocked toolkit at their disposal. They'd have a hotline to call when cravings hit, a therapist to talk them through the tough emotional triggers, and nicotine patches to soften the blow of withdrawal. But this isn't an ideal world, is it? For many smokers, these resources are out of reach. Maybe they live in a rural area with no access to cessation clinics. Maybe the cost of nicotine replacement therapies (NRTs) feels like yet another burden on top of life's many financial pressures. Or maybe they don't even know where to start looking for help.

The reality is that quitting smoking should not be a luxury afforded to the privileged few. It should be a basic human right. Everyone, regardless of their financial situation, their location, or their level of education, should have access to high-quality quit programs. Because smoking, at its core, is not just an individual health problem. It's a societal one. And society, as a whole, benefits when more people quit smoking. Fewer smokers mean lower healthcare costs, healthier workplaces, cleaner environments, and less second-hand smoke harming innocent bystanders. Everyone wins when smoking rates drop, so why wouldn't we make it as easy as possible for people to quit?

One of the most pressing arguments for making quitting programs freely available is the financial barrier to quitting smoking. On the surface, it might seem counterintuitive to say that smokers, who spend significant amounts of money on cigarettes, can't afford to quit. After all, wouldn't stopping smoking save them money in the long run? Absolutely. But here's the catch, quitting isn't free, at least not in the short term.

Nicotine patches, gum, lozenges, prescription medications, and counselling sessions can all come with a hefty price tag. For someone already stretched thin, adding these costs can feel like an impossible hurdle. And let's not forget the psychological aspect, many smokers feel trapped, believing they can't quit even if they want to. When they're already struggling, asking them to shell out more money to quit can feel like salt in the wound.

This is where government programs and public health initiatives need to step in. We need to make it as easy as possible for smokers to access the help they need, without having to weigh their financial stability against their health. Hotlines should be staffed with trained professionals who can offer advice, counselling, and resources, all free of charge. Nicotine replacement therapies, like patches and gum, should be made available at no cost to smokers looking to quit. These aren't luxuries; they're lifelines.

Imagine if every smoker who wanted to quit could walk into their local pharmacy and pick up a free quit kit. The kit could include a few weeks' supply of nicotine patches, information on local cessation support groups, and a hotline number for one-on-one counselling. Would it be expensive to roll out a program like this? Sure, initially. But the long-term savings, both in healthcare costs and in lives saved, would far outweigh the investment.

The numbers back this up. Studies show that quit programs can double, even triple, the chances of successfully quitting. The World Health Organization (WHO) has repeatedly stressed that quit support is a key part of reducing global smoking rates. In countries like the United Kingdom, where the NHS offers free stop-smoking services, the results speak for themselves. Smoking rates have steadily declined over the past decade, in part due to these widely available resources. It's a model worth replicating globally.

Let's talk about nicotine for a second. Nicotine is often painted as the villain in the smoking story, but that's only partly true. Nicotine is highly addictive, there's no arguing that, but it's not the nicotine that causes cancer or lung disease. It's the thousands of toxic chemicals in cigarette smoke that are responsible for the damage. So, when we talk about helping people quit, it's important to remember that getting rid of nicotine isn't the immediate goal. The goal is to eliminate the deadly cocktail of chemicals that cigarettes deliver. That's where nicotine replacement therapy (NRT) comes in.

NRT helps by giving smokers a small, controlled dose of nicotine without the harmful side effects of smoking. Whether it's through patches, gum, or lozenges, NRT can reduce withdrawal symptoms and cravings, making it easier for smokers to break the habit. Research consistently shows that NRT can increase the chances of quitting by 50% to 70%, especially when combined with other forms of support like counselling or behavioural therapy.

But, again, NRT is not always accessible. In many places, it's treated like any other over-the-counter product, something you pay for out of pocket. That needs to change. NRT should be subsidised or at least provided at a low cost to those who need it. And beyond NRT, there are prescription medications, like varenicline (marketed as Chantix) or bupropion (Zyban), that can help reduce cravings and withdrawal symptoms. These medications, when used correctly, have been shown to significantly improve quit rates, but they can also be expensive. Why are we putting a high price tag on something that could save the lives of over 8 million people?

In countries like the United States, where healthcare is often a barrier in itself, making these medications more affordable, or better yet, subsidised, could be a game changer. By lowering or removing the financial obstacles, we open the door for more smokers to quit, which, in turn, benefits everyone. It's a classic case of spending now to save later. Treating smoking-related illnesses costs billions every year; helping people quit costs a fraction of that.

Quitting smoking isn't just about overcoming a physical addiction; it's about unravelling the mental and emotional ties that bind someone to their cigarette habit. For many, smoking is a coping mechanism, a crutch that helps them deal with stress, anxiety, boredom, or social pressure. That's why counselling and therapy are such critical components of any quit program.

It's easy to say "just stop smoking," but anyone who has tried to quit knows it's not that simple. Smoking is often deeply intertwined with a person's identity and daily routine. Maybe it's the ritual of a cigarette with a morning coffee or the social bonding that happens during smoke breaks at work. For others, cigarettes are a way to escape or manage emotions they feel they can't handle on their own. Therapy can help smokers understand why they smoke, what triggers their cravings, and how to develop healthier coping mechanisms.

Counselling doesn't have to be a long, drawn-out process. Even a few brief sessions with a trained therapist can make a huge difference. Studies show that combining NRT or medications with counselling doubles the chances of quitting compared to using medications alone. The best part? This kind of support can be delivered in many different ways: face-to-face, over the phone, via text, or even through online platforms. There's no one-size-fits-all approach to therapy, and that flexibility is key to making sure it's accessible to everyone.

For this to work, though, we need to invest in trained professionals who understand the complexities of addiction and can offer evidence-based support. Quit lines should be staffed with experts who can guide smokers through their quit journey, offering personalised advice and encouragement. These services should be available around the clock because, let's face it, cravings don't always hit between 9 and 5. And for those who prefer face-to-face support, we need more free or low-cost cessation clinics, especially in underserved communities.

Knowledge is power, and when it comes to quitting smoking, public health campaigns play a vital role in spreading that knowledge. But it's not enough to simply tell people that smoking is bad for them, we've been doing that for decades. What we need are campaigns that focus on the benefits of quitting and highlight the resources available to help people do it.

Public health campaigns should be everywhere, on TV, in social media feeds, on billboards, in schools, and in doctors' offices. They should target different demographics, recognising that not all smokers are the same. A message that resonates with a young adult smoker might not work for a middle-aged one, and vice versa. Campaigns need to be inclusive, addressing the unique challenges faced by different groups, whether it's young people, women, ethnic minorities, or those with mental health issues.

And these campaigns shouldn't just be about the dangers of smoking; they should celebrate the successes of quitting. Highlight stories of people who've managed to break free from their addiction. Show the immediate benefits of quitting, how lungs begin to heal, how breathing becomes easier, how the risk of heart disease starts to plummet. Make quitting seem not just possible, but desirable.

But, most importantly, these campaigns should point people toward resources. It's one thing to inspire someone to quit, but it's another to give them the tools to make it happen. Every poster, every ad, every social media post should include information about free hotlines, available NRTs, and local cessation services. We need to make it crystal clear that help is out there, and it doesn't have to cost a fortune.

Community Support

The journey to quit smoking can be isolating. Even with the best quit programs and resources in place, one of the hardest aspects of quitting is feeling like you're in it alone. Smokers often build social rituals around smoking, a cigarette with colleagues during break time, sharing a smoke with friends after dinner, or simply the act of stepping outside with others for a moment of peace. When someone decides to quit, those rituals disappear, but the desire for connection doesn't.

This is where community support steps in, and why it's such a crucial part of the equation. Quitting smoking doesn't have to be a solitary endeavour. In fact, it shouldn't be. The more support a smoker has, the higher their chances of success. We need to create spaces, both physical and virtual, where ex-smokers and people who want to quit can find encouragement, share their experiences, and lean on each other when the cravings hit hard.

One of the most effective ways to support someone trying to quit smoking is through peer support groups. There's something powerful about sitting in a room (or even a virtual space) with others who know exactly what you're going through. It's the shared understanding, the lack of judgment, and the ability to talk openly about the struggles and victories that make support groups so beneficial.

Support groups can take many forms. They can be informal meetups at a local community centre, organised through healthcare providers, or even online forums where people can connect regardless of location. The key is that these groups provide a non-judgmental environment where people can share their stories, ask for advice, and offer encouragement to others on the same journey.

There's evidence to suggest that smokers who participate in group therapy or peer support groups are more likely to stay quit than those who go it alone. Why? Because quitting smoking is hard, and when you hit a rough patch, when the cravings are unbearable, when stress is pushing you toward that one cigarette, having a community that understands can make all the difference.

While professional support is essential, we can't overlook the role that family and friends play in helping someone quit smoking. Quitting isn't just a personal journey; it often affects those around the smoker. That's why it's so important to involve family and friends in the process. They need to understand the challenges the smoker is facing and how they can best support them.

But here's the catch: not everyone knows how to be supportive in the right way. Sometimes, well-meaning loved ones can inadvertently make things harder, unfortunately, I am one of those. They might nag, shame, or push too hard, which can lead to more stress and, in some cases, make a smoker feel even more tempted to light up. This is why it's crucial to educate friends and family on how to offer the right kind of support, one that's patient, compassionate, and free from judgment. By writing this book, I'm making a conscious decision to be better, to try to reach people differently in ways I probably wouldn't be able in person.

Encouraging family members to attend counselling sessions or quit groups with the smoker can be a great way to build understanding. They can learn about the psychological aspects of nicotine addiction and the emotional ups and downs that come with quitting. Armed with this knowledge, they can provide a better support system—one that's based on empathy rather than frustration.

In today's digital age, the internet has opened up new possibilities for community support. Online forums, social media groups, and quit-smoking apps offer spaces where smokers can connect with others who are trying to quit, share tips, and offer encouragement. These virtual communities have the advantage of being accessible 24/7, providing a lifeline at any time of day, especially when those late-night cravings strike.

Platforms like Reddit have thriving "quit smoking" communities, where users post daily updates, share their quitting strategies, and celebrate milestones together. The anonymity of the internet can also help smokers who may feel too ashamed or embarrassed to seek help in person. It's a safe space to ask questions, vent frustrations, and get real-time support from others who have been there.

Beyond forums, there are apps designed specifically to help people quit smoking. These apps often include features like tracking smoke-free days, calculating money saved, and even offering real-time coaching. Some apps allow users to join virtual support groups, chat with others on the same quit timeline, and participate in challenges that help keep motivation high. The beauty of these digital tools is that they're always within reach, offering encouragement at the exact moment it's needed.

The workplace is another critical environment where quitting smoking support can make a real difference. Think about it, many smokers develop their habit in the context of work. Cigarette breaks are woven into the fabric of daily office life for many smokers. But what if workplaces took a more proactive role in supporting employees who want to quit?

Employers have a vested interest in helping their staff quit smoking. Smokers, on average, take more sick days than non-smokers, are less productive due to frequent breaks, and have higher healthcare costs. By offering support programs in the workplace, employers can create a healthier, more productive environment for everyone.

Some workplaces have already started offering quitting smoking programs as part of their wellness initiatives. This can include free access to NRT, onsite counselling, or partnerships with local quit services. In some cases, employers even provide financial incentives for employees who successfully quit smoking. These programs not only help individual employees but also create a culture of health and well-being that benefits the entire workforce.

Tough Love

Now, let's shift gears. While we're all about compassion, empathy, and providing the right support to help smokers quit, there's a line that society cannot cross any longer. That line is drawn where smoking stops being a personal choice and starts being a public health hazard. The harm that smoking does to others, particularly through second-hand smoke, is too great to tolerate.

This is where tough love comes in. Yes, we need to help smokers quit, but we also need to be firm about the consequences of continuing to smoke, especially in shared spaces. Smoking is not just an individual health issue; it's a public health crisis. The evidence on second-hand smoke is irrefutable. It harms everyone who breathes it in, from children and the elderly to colleagues and complete strangers. The freedom to smoke cannot come at the cost of other people's health.

This is why public smoking bans are so essential. They're not just about protecting non-smokers from the discomfort of cigarette smoke; they're about safeguarding public health. Many countries have already implemented strict smoking bans in public places, including restaurants, bars, parks, and public transport. These laws are not just a minor inconvenience for smokers, they are a vital step in reducing exposure to toxic fumes for millions of non-smokers who have no say in the matter.

Beyond public smoking bans, we need to take a tougher stance on smoking in other shared spaces. Workplaces, schools, and public housing should all be smoke-free environments. Employers should enforce strict no-smoking policies on their premises, not just to protect non-smoking employees, but also to encourage smokers to quit.

Schools, in particular, have a duty to protect the health of their students. No child should have to walk through a cloud of cigarette smoke on their way into school. By making school grounds and surrounding areas completely smoke-free, we can set a strong example for the next generation, showing them that smoking is no longer socially acceptable.

At some point, personal responsibility has to come into play. This may sound harsh, but smokers need to understand the gravity of the harm they are inadvertently causing, not just to themselves, but to everyone around them. This is where tough love comes in. It's not about shaming or vilifying smokers; it's about being clear that their actions have real, harmful consequences.

Education is key. Smokers need to be fully informed about the impact of second-hand smoke on their loved ones, their colleagues, and the general public. But it's not enough to stop at education. There need to be consequences for those who continue to smoke in public spaces where it harms others. Hefty fines for violating public smoking bans, coupled with strong enforcement, can act as a deterrent.

In conclusion, supporting smokers in their journey to quit is a compassionate act. We know that smoking is a powerful addiction, and we must provide all the resources, tools, and community support necessary to help people break free from its grip. But at the same time, we cannot ignore the broader social responsibility to protect the health of non-smokers. The right to smoke ends where the rights of others to breathe clean air begin.

Our approach needs to be twofold: offer every possible support to help smokers quit while drawing a hard a clear line when it comes to the health and safety of others. Through quit programs, community support, and tough love, we can work toward a future where smoking no longer poses a threat to anyone, neither the smoker nor the people around them.

Chapter 10 | The End of the Road: A Future Without Cigarettes

A brief summary

It's been a long, winding road. Decades of cigarette smoke trailing through our lives, infiltrating homes, businesses, schools, parks, and even the most intimate spaces where we seek comfort. This is the road we call the *Cancer Highway*, a destructive path that has claimed the lives of millions, leaving behind a legacy of suffering, disease, and death. But today, as we stand at the crossroads, we must make a choice: to continue down this path or to create a future where cigarettes are no longer a part of our story.

For too long, smoking has been a vehicle speeding towards a cliff, and for too long, society has watched it drive recklessly toward inevitable disaster. We've known the truth about cigarettes for generations, the way they lead to heart disease, cancer, respiratory illness, and untimely death. We've seen the toll they've taken on families, friendships, and communities. Yet, despite the mountain of evidence, cigarettes have remained on the shelves, legal, accessible, and somehow still socially acceptable in some circles.

But why? How have we allowed this to continue? The answer lies not in ignorance but in apathy and in the sheer force of the tobacco industry's grip on public policy, culture, and economics. Cigarettes have woven themselves into the fabric of society, becoming more than just a habit, they're a commodity, a symbol, a deeply ingrained addiction. But it doesn't have to be this way. The *Cancer Highway* doesn't need to remain open. We have the power to shut it down and create a world where cigarettes belong to the past, alongside other toxic substances we've wisely eradicated from daily life.

Smoking is nothing short of a journey, a perilous one. From the first puff, most people are unaware of where they are headed. They're drawn in by the allure of rebellion, social acceptance, stress relief, or simply the influence of friends and family who smoke. Some are even seduced by glorified portrayals of smoking in media. But this journey, for all its perceived benefits, is a one-way ticket to destruction.

Imagine driving down a highway without rules, smooth roads, fast lanes, no visible dangers at first. It feels liberating. For many smokers, this is how the habit begins. The first few cigarettes don't seem to bring immediate harm. But like any highway, there are signs along the way, these signs at first appeared inviting, but these warnings were designed to look like that. Up-close, these are warnings that show the journey ahead isn't as smooth as it first appeared. Maybe it's a lingering cough that doesn't go away, shortness of breath after climbing the stairs, or stained teeth. Maybe it's noticing a loved one struggling with chronic health issues brought on by smoking. The signs are dismissive at first, but they become harder to ignore as the journey continues.

As you travel further along this *Cancer Highway*, the consequences become more severe. Heart disease, strokes, emphysema, and, of course, the dreaded word: cancer. Lung cancer, oral cancer, throat cancer, cigarettes are merciless in their ability to attack nearly every part of the body. And it's not just the smoker who suffers. There is no riding alone in this highway, smokers will always bring passengers with them, family, friends, co-workers, even strangers, they are forced to inhale the toxic fumes, their own health sacrificed because of someone else's choice. The road is not just for the smoker; it's a highway that pulls in innocent bystanders.

But the end of this road is where the real tragedy lies. It's a precipice, a cliff that leads to immense suffering. Lung cancer is one of the deadliest forms of cancer, and for many, it's a death sentence. Those who reach this stage often face years of pain, surgeries, chemotherapy, radiation, and the unbearable emotional toll that comes with knowing their life is being cut short. The lucky ones may quit before this point, but even then, the damage is often done. The scars of smoking, both physical and emotional, remain.

The *Cancer Highway* is not just a personal journey, it's a societal one. Every year, millions of people travel down this path, their lives dictated by an addiction that profits only the tobacco industry while devastating public health. But it doesn't have to be this way. This is a road that can be closed. There are exits in the form of quitting programs, support systems, and legislation that can steer people away from this dangerous path. The road can, and must, be shut down for good.

We cannot sit idly by and allow this highway to remain open. Every year, more lives are lost, more families are torn apart, more children are exposed to second-hand smoke. This is not just an individual problem, it is a public health crisis, and it demands action from every one of us.

We need to challenge the status quo and demand stronger measures to curb smoking. The first step is supporting stricter bans on cigarettes and tobacco products. Many countries have made progress by banning smoking in public places, but this is not enough. We need comprehensive bans that make it harder for people to access cigarettes in the first place. This includes higher taxes on tobacco products, which have been shown to reduce smoking rates, particularly among young people. The higher the price, the less attractive smoking becomes, especially to those who are just starting the habit.

But taxes and bans are just part of the solution. We must also push for more aggressive anti-smoking legislation that goes beyond regulation and aims for total eradication. This means advocating for laws that hold the tobacco industry accountable for the harm they've caused. For too long, Big Tobacco has operated with impunity, raking in profits while knowingly selling a product that kills. They must be forced to pay for the damage they've done, through fines, lawsuits, and stringent regulations that make it nearly impossible for them to continue their business as usual.

As individuals, we can also play a critical role in helping those around us quit smoking. Quitting is not easy, it's a process that often takes multiple attempts and a lot of support. But it's not impossible, and with the right tools, people can break free from nicotine addiction. We need to encourage our friends and family to seek help, whether that's through quitting programs, nicotine replacement therapy, or simply offering emotional support. For some, quitting may seem like an insurmountable task, but with the right resources and a strong support system, it can be done.

Finally, we need to raise our voices against the normalization of smoking in media and culture. Smoking should not be glamorised in films, television shows, or advertisements. It's time to challenge the idea that smoking is cool or rebellious. It's not. It's deadly. By speaking out and pushing back against the portrayal of smoking as something desirable, we can help shift public perception and make smoking a relic of the past.

A Vision for the Future: A World Without Cigarettes

Imagine a world where cigarettes no longer exist. Where the smell of smoke doesn't linger in public places, where children don't have to grow up watching their parents puff away at cigarettes, and where the air is clean, free of the toxins that have plagued us for decades. This is not a far-fetched dream, it's a reality that is within our grasp, if we are willing to fight for it.

A smoke-free world would be a healthier, happier place for all of us. Think about the impact on public health, fewer cases of lung cancer, heart disease, and respiratory illnesses. Hospitals would see a reduction in patients suffering from smoking-related diseases, freeing up resources to tackle other pressing health issues. The financial burden on healthcare systems would be significantly reduced, saving billions in medical costs and lost productivity. Governments could redirect those funds toward education, infrastructure, and social services, improving the quality of life for everyone.

Future generations could grow up without the shadow of cigarettes looming over them. Children would no longer be exposed to second-hand smoke, which has been proven to cause serious health problems, including asthma, respiratory infections, and even sudden infant death syndrome (SIDS). Young people wouldn't be tempted to pick up the habit because cigarettes would be viewed as a relic of the past, something dangerous, outdated, and completely unnecessary.

We've done it before. Think of how society has moved on from other toxic substances like lead in gasoline, asbestos in building materials, or radium pills that were once sold as health products. These substances were once commonplace, considered essential or even beneficial, until we realised the immense harm they were causing. And once we knew the truth, we took action. We banned them, regulated them, and made them illegal. Now, they are seen for what they are, dangerous, poisonous, and unthinkable in modern society.

Cigarettes are no different. They are a product that serves no positive purpose. They kill, they maim, and they destroy lives. In the future, smoking will be viewed just as we now view those other dangerous substances, something that was once accepted but is now seen as a tragic mistake. The question is, which side of history do you want to be on? Will you be part of the generation that finally said enough is enough? Or will you stand by and let this deadly product continue to claim lives?

The *Cancer Highway* has only one end, a precipice of pain, suffering, and injustice. But here's the truth: it doesn't have to end that way. There is a stop, a chance to turn off this road before it's too late. It won't be easy, the breaks in this vehicle-of-doom are hidden, hard to access, and they are designed to be that way. For many, quitting smoking feels like an impossible task, and for society, dismantling the tobacco industry may seem like an uphill battle. But it is possible. With the right combination of individual effort, collective action, and strong legislation, we can make this change.

We owe it to future generations to end this highway before it claims more lives that never signed up for the ride. We owe it to the millions of people who have suffered and died because of smoking. We owe it to ourselves to live in a world that is free from the toxic grip of cigarettes.

This journey toward a smoke-free future won't happen overnight, but the seeds of change have already been planted. Activists, health organisations, and governments around the world are working tirelessly to reduce smoking rates, hold the tobacco industry accountable, and protect public health. Their work is critical, and we must join them in this fight. We must lend our voices to their cause, support their efforts, and push for the stronger measures that are needed to finally rid the world of cigarettes.

The *Cancer Highway* must end here, before it takes more lives that never signed up for the ride. Only the smoker can unlock the door for the passengers that are taking along this road without their consent, only the smoker is capable to stop this vehicle, to steer it towards the hard-to-see but a very much real exit path. We as society stand at the crossroads. The choice is ours. Will we continue down this deadly road, or will we own up and create a future where cigarettes no longer have a place in our world? The answer seems clear. Now, it's up to all of us to make it a reality.

I WANT TO QUIT

I f you read this far is because you want to make a difference, and despite my harsh approaches to the habit, we as humans must look out for each other, I want you to get better so we can all get better together. Quitting smoking is one of the hardest battles a person can fight, but it's also one of the most rewarding. When we look at the toll tobacco takes on our health, not to mention the burden it places on our families and society, the urgency to quit becomes clear. It's not just about saving your own life, though that's a pretty good reason, it's also about reducing the impact on those around you, including children, partners, and co-workers, who are often the silent victims of second-hand smoke.

Fortunately, many resources are available to help smokers quit, and organisations are tirelessly advocating for stronger laws to protect public health. Whether you're in the U.S. or the UK, or another country entirely, the path to quitting is supported by many who are dedicated to this fight. Below, we'll explore some of the most effective resources available for those looking to quit smoking, along with advocacy groups pushing for stricter regulations. Please make good use of the internet search of your choice and take that next step to recovery.

Quitting Smoking Resources in the United States

In the United States, smoking cessation resources are both plentiful and diverse. Here are some of the key programs and tools that can support your journey:

1. Smokefree.gov (https://www.smokefree.gov/)

One of the most comprehensive online resources for quitting is **Smoke-free.gov**, a government-backed initiative. Smokefree.gov offers free quit plans, tips, and expert support through phone, text, and chat services. Their tools are personalised based on your quitting needs, and they offer tailored advice for different groups, such as veterans, teens, and women who are pregnant. For those who prefer mobile support, the Smokefree app is a valuable tool that offers 24/7 motivation and guidance.

2. 1-800-QUIT-NOW

This national helpline provides free coaching and support to anyone who's ready to quit smoking. Call **1-800-QUIT-NOW** to get connected with a counsellor who can help you create a plan tailored to your needs. They also offer free resources such as nicotine patches or gum, depending on your location. It's a hands-on service with real people ready to guide you through each stage of quitting.

3. Truth Initiative (https://truthinitiative.org/)

Truth Initiative is known for its hard-hitting campaigns aimed at youth and young adults, but they also provide extensive resources to help people quit. Their innovative text messaging programs like "This Is Quitting" offer support to young smokers trying to quit vaping or smoking traditional cigarettes. Truth Initiative is also heavily involved in advocacy, pushing for stricter regulations on tobacco products.

4. American Lung Association (https://www.lung.org/)

The **American Lung Association** provides various tools and programs to help people quit smoking, including Freedom From Smoking, an evidence-based program that has helped thousands of Americans quit. Their website also offers extensive educational materials, and they advocate for stronger tobacco control laws.

Quitting Smoking Resources in the United Kingdom

In the UK, the government and health organisations have developed a wide array of tools to support smokers who want to quit. From free stop-smoking services to digital tools, here are some of the key resources:

1. NHS Smokefree (https://www.nhs.uk/better-health/quit-smoking/)

NHS Smokefree is the National Health Service's free quitting programme. It provides smokers with a wealth of information, support, and tools to help them quit. The website offers free personal quit plans, access to free stop-smoking services, and advice on the use of nicotine replacement therapies (NRT) like patches and gum. There is also the NHS Smokefree app, which helps track your progress and provides motivation along the way.

2. Quitline

Quitline is a phone service available in the UK that connects smokers with trained advisors who provide one-on-one support to help you quit. You can contact the service by calling 0300 123 1044. It's an easy and accessible way to get direct advice from experts.

3. ASH (Action on Smoking and Health - https://ash.org.uk/)

ASH UK is one of the leading advocacy groups in the United Kingdom, working to reduce the harm caused by tobacco through public health campaigns and policy changes. ASH provides information on quitting smoking, and their resources often focus on protecting children and young people from the harmful effects of smoking. If you are looking for broader information on the tobacco epidemic or wish to get involved in advocacy, ASH is a vital organisation to explore.

4. British Lung Foundation (https://www.blf.org.uk/)

The British Lung Foundation offers support for smokers who want to quit, with advice on how to use cessation aids like patches, gum, or prescription medications. They also provide guidance on how to access local quit-smoking services, including help for those with chronic lung conditions who need more tailored assistance in quitting.

Advocacy Groups and Movements Fighting for Stricter Laws

Fighting the tobacco industry is no easy feat, but there are organisations around the world working to push for tougher laws to protect public health and reduce smoking rates. Whether you want to support these movements or get involved, here are some leading advocacy groups in the U.S. and UK:

United States

- **Campaign for Tobacco-Free Kids**: One of the largest organisations advocating for stronger tobacco control laws in the U.S. The Campaign for Tobacco-Free Kids works at both state and federal levels to push for policies that limit tobacco marketing, increase cigarette taxes, and ban flavoured products that target young people. (https://www.tobaccofreekids.org/)
- **American Cancer Society (ACS)**: While the ACS is primarily known for funding cancer research, they also have a strong advocacy arm focused on tobacco control. The ACS's Cancer Action Network advocates for smoke-free laws, tax hikes on tobacco, and other measures to reduce smoking rates. (https://www.fightcancer.org/)

United Kingdom

- **ASH UK (Action on Smoking and Health)**: As mentioned earlier, ASH UK is one of the most active groups in the UK working to promote policies that prevent smoking, especially among young people. They are key players in lobbying for legislative changes and stricter tobacco regulations.
- **Fresh – Smoke Free North East**: This regional initiative in the North East of England is dedicated to making the area the first truly smoke-free region in the country. They work with local communities and policymakers to advocate for stricter tobacco control and provide resources for quitting.

Finding Resources in Other Countries

If you're outside the U.S. or UK, don't worry – most countries have similar quit-smoking resources and advocacy groups. The World Health Organization (WHO) is a great starting point to find global smoking cessation resources. Their Tobacco Free Initiative works with countries around the world to implement smoking control policies and provides resources for people looking to quit.

https://www.who.int/initiatives/tobacco-free-initiative

You can also contact your local health authorities or search for quit-smoking programs in your country. Many countries offer free national quitlines, government-sponsored websites, and regional tobacco control organisations that can help you quit.

Another helpful tip is to visit local pharmacies, where quit-smoking products like patches, gum, and lozenges are often available, and pharmacists can offer advice on where to seek support. Additionally, many global health organisations, like the American Cancer Society and the International Union Against Tuberculosis and Lung Disease, have branches or partnerships worldwide that work to support smokers trying to quit.

Final Thoughts

Quitting smoking is one of the most courageous and impactful decisions you can make, not only for your health but for those around you. Resources and support are more accessible than ever, no matter where you are in the world. The key is to take that first step, whether it's picking up the phone to call a quitline or visiting a website to create your personalised quit plan.

If you're motivated by the broader fight against tobacco, consider getting involved with advocacy groups that push for stronger laws. Every voice count, especially when we're up against an industry that profits from addiction and sickness. The battle against tobacco is far from over, but with the right support, it's one we can win.